"I had surgery for carpal tunnel syndrome, but still had tremendous pain in the wrist, arm and elbow. Kate has taught me self-correcting techniques to relieve the stress and tension by realigning the wrist and elbow that I can do as needed, diminishing the pain, enabling me to get through the day and do my job. As a result of Kate's massage therapy and pain relief training I will not undergo surgery on my elbow or on my other wrist. There are not enough words in the human language to express my gratitude. I only wish I had found you sooner."

Cynthia Weaver
Administrative Secretary, County of San Diego
Santee, California

"A method that is sure to help anyone who uses it as directed."

Dr. John Thie, DC.
President of TOUCH FOR HEALTH

"A brief encounter in a restaurant with Kate Montgomery corrected a new carpal tunnel problem for me—a recurrence of pain and dysfunction after five surgeries. When Kate corrected my elbow and wrist joint, I received immediate relief from the loss of touch I had been experiencing! Now that I understand the physiology of the problem, I can use her simple and easy exercises to strengthen my hands and self-correct this problem if it recurs."

Patti Graff, Writer
Vista, California

"Kate's Carpal Tunnel program will decrease office visits and overall cost of therapy and the patient is able to return to work faster."

William Lerner, DC.
Del Mar, California

" I met Kate Montgomery at a conference in 1992 and she demonstrated a self-help method for the treatment of symptoms of Carpal Tunnel Syndrome. I found her method to be effective and it really helps. Kate's Carpal Tunnel method is safe, cost effective and eliminates the need for surgical intervention in most cases. The exercises are simple and easy to do, with minimal amount of instruction. The corrective techniques are designed to be done anywhere. It is an answer to decreasing the workers compensation problem and getting employees back to work with minimal or no work time lost. I highly recommend this program."

Warren Jacobs, MD.
Family Practice for over 30 years
Escondido, California

"If you can imagine a whole year of dealing with increasing pain, able to do less and less, and terribly anxious about not being able to continue my career in music, the relief, and the new hope that this pain-free state engendered, was very dramatic. I felt overwhelmed with gratitude toward this knowledge woman. I have learned the reasons for the pain, and that knowledge has strengthened my resolve to take the corrective healing measures which Kate has taught me. It all makes sense—and Kate is showing me the way!"

Sheila Sterling
Principle Harpist, San Diego Symphony
and San Diego Opera for 25 years

"I have lived with Carpal Tunnel Syndrome and have taken my daily dose of drugs to relieve the pain in my hands. Three years ago I met Kate Montgomery and what a difference she made in my life. She taught me how to do self-corrective techniques to prevent CTS and when I feel it reoccurring, I can nip it in the bud. I get instant relief from the pain. I don't dread going to work or doing my outside activities. I feel great and I feel creative all the time! Thanks to Kate, I am now comfortable in my workplace and my life."

Judy Hughes, Graphic Designer
and Professional Dog Groomer
San Diego, California

"Having been a big band drummer for over 50 years, the trauma received from constant timekeeping on drum heads, cymbals, and especially from heavy rim shots, created a pain in my hands and wrists. Kate's carpal tunnel self-corrective exercises have eliminated the pain and discomfort immediately. These can be done in just a few seconds, even while sitting on the bandstand. My hands are always strong and playing is effortless now!"

Jim Janecki- Big Band Drummer, Chicago 15
San Diego, California

CARPAL TUNNEL SYNDROME

Prevention & Treatment

A NonSurgical, Drug Free Approach

The Repetitive Strain Injury of the Wrist and Hand

by Kate Montgomery
Certified Sports Massage Therapist

WORD OF CAUTION: Trauma to the hand and loss of its function is a serious matter. If after trying these simple techniques, no relief is evident, see a chiropractor specializing in applied kinesiology or a physician specializing in the hand for more indepth tests.

SPORTS TOUCH ® PUBLISHING
P.O. Box 221074
San Diego, CA 92192-1074
Copyright 1992, 1993, 1994
ISBN 1-878069-35-7
"SPORTS TOUCH®" is registered with the U.S. Patent and Trademark office.

First Edition 1992
Second Edition 1993
Third Edition 1994

Contents

Foreword

Long before writing this book, I read many articles on the subject of Carpal Tunnel Syndrome (CTS), the Repetitive Strain Injury (RSI) of the wrist and hand. Throughout my travels in this country and abroad, RSI is the number one worker's compensation claim. Due to recurring injuries, many people have missed work or even lost their jobs and feel surgery is the only recourse. But, surgery is a temporary solution and, in many cases, fails to eradicate CTS. Most people have tried physical therapy, acupuncture and/or massage and still have had only minimal relief. These modalities should be implemented but not until the structure has been realigned. I am concerned that people do not understand the basic definition of Carpal Tunnel Syndrome or RSI and are being misinformed and misguided on how it should be properly treated.

My book is not a cure for Carpal Tunnel Syndrome or RSI but a preventive and self-treatment program that any individual can incorporate into their daily lifestyle and schedule. My instructions and techniques bring the bodys' structure and muscles back into balance. The body is not a robot and cannot function that way. It moves out of balance daily due to the mental and physical stress of normal activities. The inception and growth of the computer age has brought RSI to the forefront. It is my intention to provide helpful information and insight about this disease of the nineties.

I sincerely hope that this book and the program I have developed offers relief from the pain suffered by those with Carpal Tunnel Syndrome or RSI.

KATE MONTGOMERY
President, Sports Touch®

Introduction

In the 1990s, Carpal Tunnel Syndrome has become the surgery of the decade. This is unfortunate because not only is the operation very expensive, but it causes loss of the use of the hand for two to six months with no guarantee of post-surgical improvement. And, I am sorry to say, in most cases pain and dysfunction returns due to a build-up of scar tissue in the surgical area. Anyone who uses his/her hands and wrists and bends the elbows may be at risk of developing Carpal Tunnel Syndrome.

In today's world, many careers create stress on our elbows and wrists—from the very technically advanced to the most routine job. People in occupations that involve forceful or repetitive use of the hands are at risk to develop Carpal Tunnel Syndrome. A study in Rochester, Minnesota, suggests that women are developing Carpal Tunnel Syndrome at a greater rate than men—outnumbering them three to one.

Carpal tunnel trauma to the hand can be caused by many factors. Are you a waiter who carries heavy trays, hyperextending your hand? Do you scrub floors while leaning on the opposite hand? Are you a grocery clerk who repeatedly waves your hand over an electronic eye? Are you a computer programmer, baker, golfer, tennis player, a carpenter, a mechanic, a weightlifter, a musician, a massage therapist, a student who carries heavy books? The list goes on and on. All these careers, and more, can lead to Carpal Tunnel Syndrome.

Short of stopping the activity that aggravates the condition, Carpal Tunnel Syndrome can be prevented or improved by alleviating muscular tension through a health maintenance program and redesigning tools, workstations and job tasks.

Prevention is the key to strong and stable joints. A health maintenance program of chiropractic and massage therapy along with a daily exercise program, insures and prevents the recurrence Carpal Tunnel Syndrome.

What Is Carpal Tunnel Syndrome?

I.

Carpal Tunnel Syndrome is an entrapment and compression of the median nerve due to a structural and postural misalignment brought on by the overworked and overstrained muscles of the arms and hands, leading to a muscle strength problem. Persons who perform continuous repetitive movements are at higher risk to develop CTS. ▶

What is this Ailment?

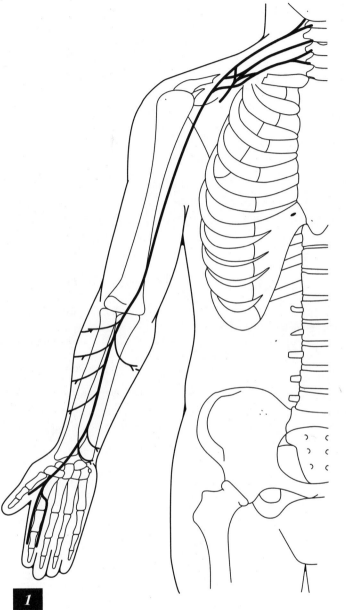

1

A median nerve entrapment can develop at many locations—from the vertebral joints in the neck through the shoulder joint, descending to the elbow joint and ending with the final distortion and pain in the wrist and hand. (*Fig. 1*)

2 SIGNS AND SYMPTOMS OF CARPAL TUNNEL SYNDROME

1. Loss of the sense of touch.

2. Tingling and numbness in the hand and fingers.

3. Pain at night in the shoulder while sleeping.

4. Pain in the elbow area.

5. Swelling in the wrist area.

6. Loss of grip strength in the hand.

7. Pain in the wrist joint when the wrist joint is in hyperextension or hyperflexion.

8. Increased occurrence of dropping objects.

9. A burning sensation in the wrist and hand area.

10. Are you unable to unscrew a jar cap?

11. Is it hard to brush your hair?

12. Have you had to give up doing things with your hands because it hurts too much?

13. In extreme cases, atrophy of the forearm and hand muscles. (Atrophy is the tightening and shrinking of the muscles from nonuse which decreases movement and flexibility.)

14. Women: Any fluctuations in hormone levels that induces swelling or bloating, such as in pregnancy, PMS, and menopause, may aggravate Carpal Tunnel Syndrome. Consult with your doctor.

15. A person with long standing diabetes could suffer from peripheral vascular disease, which could lead to muscular myopathy. Consult with your doctor.

16. Any sustained trauma to the hands can cause damage to the nerves, tendons and muscles.

You may have Carpal Tunnel Syndrome!

ANATOMY OF THE HAND

The hand is comprised of eight carpal bones, five metacarpal bones and fourteen phalanges.

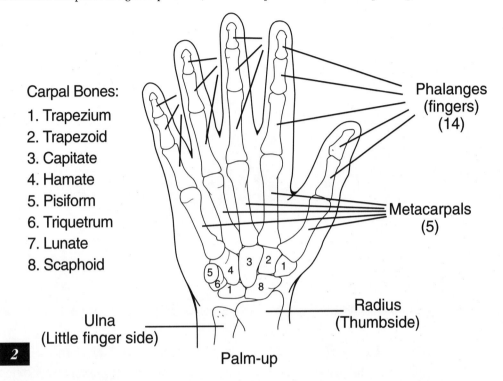

Carpal Bones:
1. Trapezium
2. Trapezoid
3. Capitate
4. Hamate
5. Pisiform
6. Triquetrum
7. Lunate
8. Scaphoid

Phalanges
(fingers)
(14)

Metacarpals
(5)

Radius
(Thumbside)

Ulna
(Little finger side)

2

Palm-up

6 ▶

As pictured in Fig. 2A (the hand, palm side-up), there are four bones that form the carpal tunnel. They are the Hook of Hamate, Pisiform, Navicular Tuberosity and the Tubercle of Trapezium.

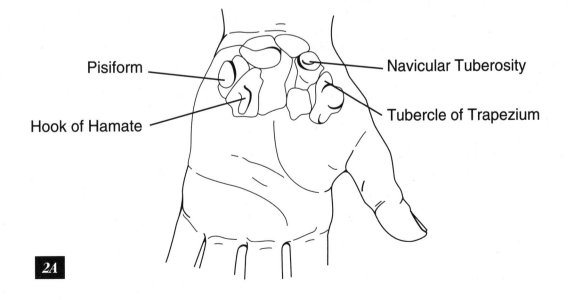

Pisiform

Navicular Tuberosity

Hook of Hamate

Tubercle of Trapezium

2A

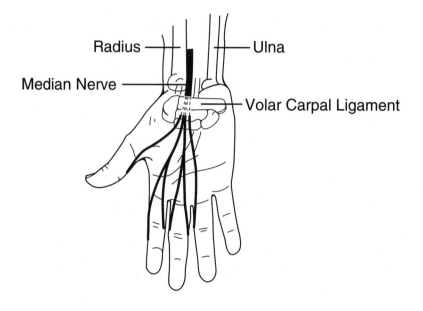

Radius ——

—— Ulna

Median Nerve ——

—— Volar Carpal Ligament

3

The volar carpal ligament runs between the four bony prominences and forms a fibrous sheath. Transported through this tunnel is the median nerve and the finger flexor tendons of the forearm and hand.

When the arm bones (radius and ulna) become splayed apart due to a misalignment of the elbow joint, a weakness develops in the wrist muscle, Pronator Quadratus. (*Fig. 4*) As the radius and ulna move apart, the volar carpal ligament becomes stretched, applying pressure on the median nerve and the finger flexor tendons of the forearm and hand causing pain, muscle weakness and narrowing the tunnel pathway. (*Fig. 3*)

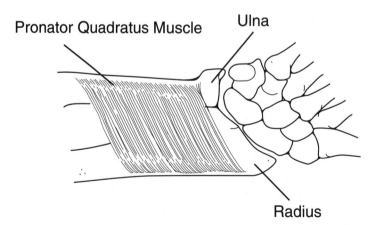

Pronator Quadratus Muscle

Ulna

Radius

4

4 MUSCLES USED FOR GRIP STRENGTH

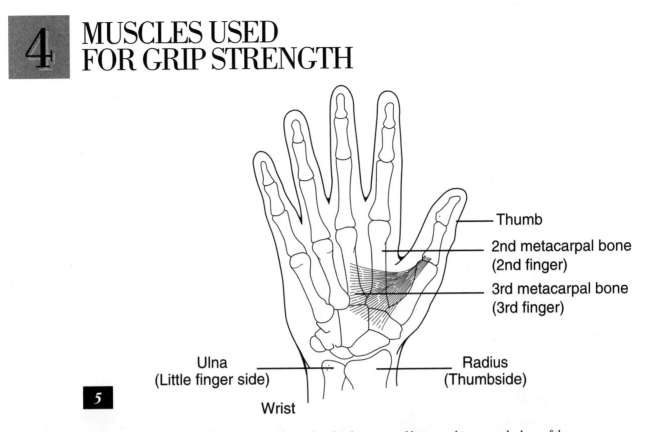

— Thumb

— 2nd metacarpal bone (2nd finger)

— 3rd metacarpal bone (3rd finger)

Ulna (Little finger side)

Radius (Thumbside)

Wrist

5

The Adductor Pollicis muscle originates at the 2nd and 3rd metacarpal bones and inserts at the base of the thumb. The action of this muscle is to draw the thumb toward the little finger and assist with the grip of the hand. (*Fig. 5*)

The Opponens Digiti Minimi originates in a fibrous band covering the carpal tunnel at the wrist and the hamate bone on the ulnar side of the wrist and inserts at the ulnar side of the 5th metacarpal bone, (little finger.) The action of this muscle is to rotate and draw the little finger toward the thumb. It too assists with the grip of the hand. (*Fig. 6*)

8 ▶

What Is Carpal Tunnel Syndrome?

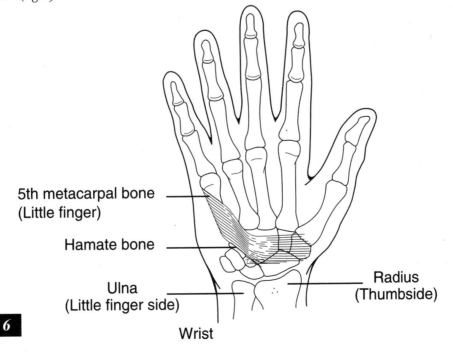

5th metacarpal bone (Little finger)

Hamate bone

Ulna (Little finger side)

Radius (Thumbside)

Wrist

6

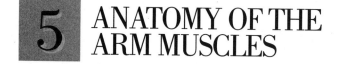

5 ANATOMY OF THE ARM MUSCLES

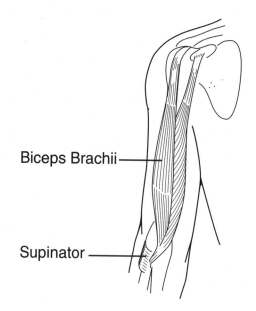

Biceps Brachii—

Supinator—

7

9 ▶

What Is
Carpal
Tunnel
Syndrome?

The muscles in the forearm that are responsible for the movement of pronation (rotate inward) and supination (rotate outward) originate at the elbow joint. When the forearm muscles become over-worked and over-strained from constant repetition, the pronator and supinator muscles develop trigger points (refer to glossary). The muscles, in time, become less flexible and mobile, tight and are painful to touch. Misalignment of the elbow joint will increase with the repetitive stress and tension on these muscles. The compromised median nerve as it passes through the elbow joint, produces pain in the elbow area. This is commonly called tendenitis or "tennis elbow." Tendenitis is a precursor to carpal tunnel syndrome. Structural realignment, trigger point release and massage will free up this joint, eliminating pain in the muscles. (*Fig. 7 & 8*)

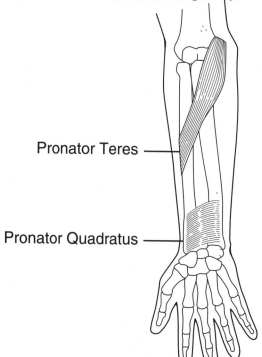

Pronator Teres—

Pronator Quadratus—

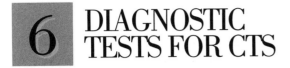
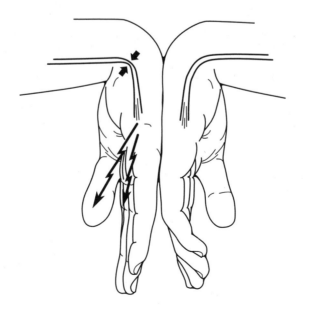

9

Diagnostic tests such as the Tinel test, (tapping the volar carpal ligament over the median nerve to elicit a pain response) *(Fig.9)*, Phalens test, (extreme hyperextension and hyperflexion of the wrist) *(Fig.10)*, and Applied Kinesiology techniques (muscle monitoring for muscle weakness in the hand) can help to determine Carpal Tunnel Syndrome.

10 ▶

What Is
Carpal
Tunnel
Syndrome?

10

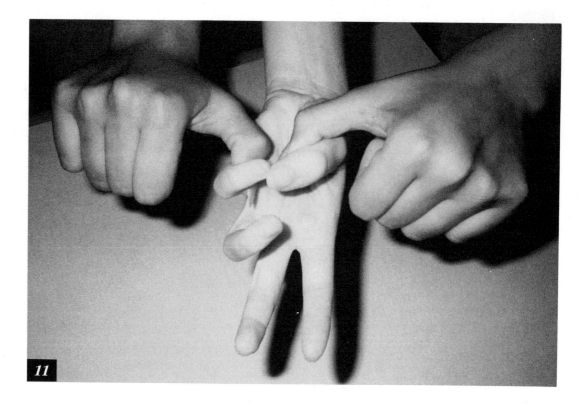

11

"Applied Kinesiology is a system which evaluates our structural, chemical and mental aspects. It employs muscle testing with other standard methods of diagnosis, nutrition, manipulation, acupressure, exercise and education to restore balance and maintain well being throughout life."

As a massage therapist, I use these techniques to monitor muscle strength and bilateral balance. It is a unique tool used in the healing arts to accentuate healing and recovery. (*Fig. 11*)

*Definition from the International College of Applied Kinesiology.

To date, almost everyone I have screened has Carpal Tunnel Syndrome in one form or another. You may not know you have it because you don't have any pain or symptoms. By using applied kinesiology techniques, muscle monitoring, to determine the muscular weakness of the thumb muscles (Abductor Pollicis Brevis, Adductor Pollicis, Flexor Pollicis Brevis and Opponens Pollicis) and the little finger muscles (Abductor Digiti Minimi, Flexor Digiti Minimi, and Opponens Digiti Minimi), you can determine if you have Carpal Tunnel Syndrome. Muscle monitoring determines the loss of strength of the thumb and the little finger muscles that help to make up the grip strength of the hand, the misalignment of the carpal bones (hand bones) and the elbow joint. In my research, I have observed that a person can change his/her posture in the neck and shoulder area (Example: Sit up straight and pull the shoulders back), uncompromise the wrist by wearing a wrist brace or placing a support under the wrist to guard against hyperflexing the wrist, bending the wrist backwards. (Ex. A three-quarter inch pad in front of the keyboard. Pg. 53.)

The one joint that we can not protect and the most ignored is the elbow. The elbow joint is in constant motion and has the most stress applied to it. Most of us don't do any kind of exercises to strengthen our arm tendons and muscles. An example is sitting at a computer, eight hours a day/five days a week, the elbow is bent at a 90° angle. Even if you have correct posture, an ergonomically correct workstation, your wrist is in a neutral position, the elbow joint is compromised. My theory is that the weight of the bones puts stress on the tendons that support and hold the joint together. The constant repetition of a specific motion will cause the muscles of the forearm to become tight, sore and fatigue from overuse. Trigger points activate when the muscles go into spasm. When this occurs, the tightness of the tendons and muscles put stress on the bones, pulling the bones out of alignment. The constant, day-to-day movement of the finger, hand, and arm muscles puts stress on the elbow joint when it is held in one position for a number of hours, or when there is direct weight on the elbow and wrist joints. My conception of the whole arm includes the micromovement of the tendons, muscles and nerves. The micromovement of the elbow and wrist joints is undetected by an x-ray exam.

The only way to detect a change in the nerve conduction other than electromyography, is through applied kinesiology. Muscle monitoring can show immediate change in the muscular strength of the hand muscles and detect the possible misalignment of the bones involved in the impingement of the median nerve.

What people and employers don't understand is that it is not only occupations with repetitive motion that cause Carpal Tunnel Syndrome or RSI, normal everyday life is also a cause. Only since the computer age, has Repetitive Strain Injury come to our attention and become the disease of the '90s.

Once CTS or RSI is determined, you can restore vital energy and neural sensation, rebuild strength in your hand, improve on surgical results, relieve existing problems, and begin a ongoing preventive program for Carpal Tunnel Syndrome.

In Most Cases, The Results Are Immediate!

When you correct Carpal Tunnel Syndrome, you will feel re-emergence of your sense of touch and strength in your hand. After performing the restorative movements, the tendons and muscles around your elbow and wrist joint may feel sore the next day. That's because your elbow bones will be back in the correct alignment, as will be the tendons and muscles that support and hold the joints together. With the aid of massage therapy, the muscle soreness, tendinitis, trigger points and pain will disappear.

Correction can be very simple in most cases and SURGERY CAN BE AVOIDED.

Muscle
Monitoring

II.

The science of Applied Kinesiology or commonly called muscle monitoring is a system that is a holistic approach to balancing the vital energy of the body to increase performance and recovery within the body.

Muscle Monitoring is a unique and immediate method of assessing what is "out of balance" in the body. When the body shifts, compensation and misalignment take place. When you sit and perform repetitive movements for hours, the stress on the muscles is comparable to running a marathon.

If you do not allow the muscles to rest and receive massage therapy to encourage muscular recovery, the body will eventually wear down and become vulnerable to injury.

Muscle Monitoring is a tool, when used on a regular basis along with other modes of therapy can prevent both injury and the deterioration of the body. ▶

MUSCLE MONITORING TECHNIQUES

If in both tests, the fingers come apart easily, you may have a misalignment of the bones in the wrist and elbow joint, with possible misalignment in the shoulder and neck area. The latter depends on if you have had a previous back, shoulder or neck injury (ie. whiplash) or positioned your body in an incorrect posture for many years. This could lead to a loss of nerve conductivity and muscular strenght in the hands. This is a sign you may have Carpal Tunnel Syndrome or a nerve conduction disorder involving other nerves of the upper body.

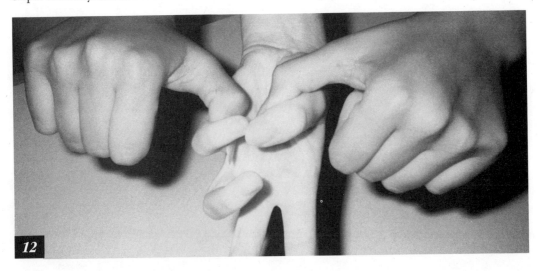

To determine if you have Carpal Tunnel Syndrome:

Place the pads of your thumb and little finger together, palm side-up, and have a friend try to pull the thumb and little finger apart. (*Fig. 12*) Place the pads of your thumb and little finger together, palm side-down, and have a friend try to pull the thumb and little finger apart. (*Fig. 13*)

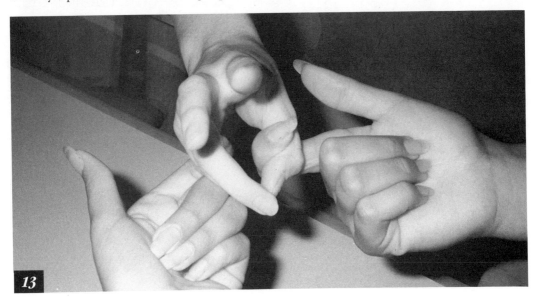

*For more information on Applied Kinesiology, refer to *Applied Kinesiology* by David S. Walter and Touch For Health by John Thie, D.C.

GRIP STRENGTH ASSESSMENT OF THE HAND

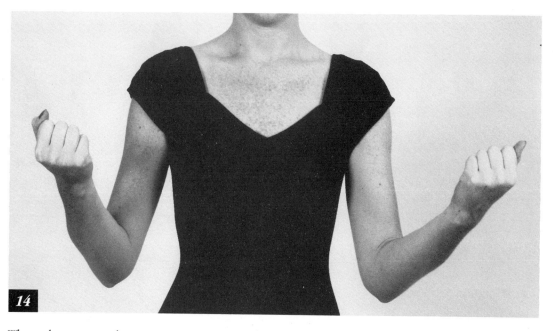

14

When a dynamometer that measures your grip strength is unavailable, a simple method of squeezing your fists together can help you determine the change in your grip strength. Squeeze your fists firmly together, give yourself a number (1-10) that you feel measures your grip strength. How strong do you feel? Perform the corrections as indicated in Chapter III. Squeeze your fists together to see if your grip strength has improved. You should feel an improvement in grip strength. Correct one arm at a time and compare the difference in grip strength between the two hands. Remember, you can repeat the corrections as much as you need to achieve the desired results. (*Fig. 14*)

Corrective Techniques

III.

The CTS techniques introduce you to a practical and functional program of self-correction, exercises and stretches, that can be incorporated into your lifestyle, anytime and anywhere. It is a self-help program designed for the mobility, support and stabilization of the muscles and joints of the arm. ▶

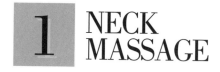

1 NECK MASSAGE

This relaxes the neck muscles and increases flexibility, nerve function and blood circulation.

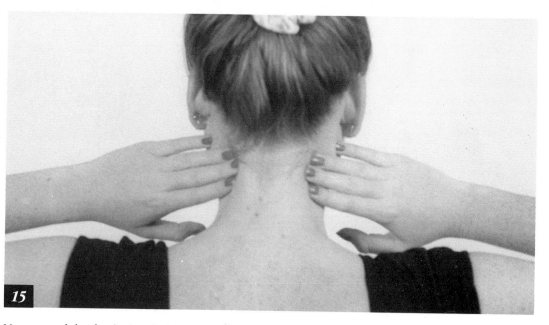

15

Massage gently but firmly along both sides of the neck vertebrae. (*Fig. 15*) Do this for approximately one-five minutes. Then gently traction upward at the base of the skull. (*Fig. 16*)

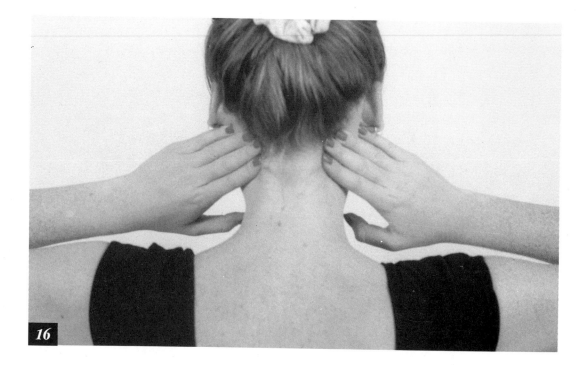

16

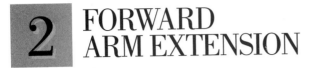

2 FORWARD ARM EXTENSION

This realigns the elbow joint in the forward line. Perform the forward extension three times on each arm. Repeat exercises on the opposite arm. This exercise can be done as often as needed to achieve desired results.

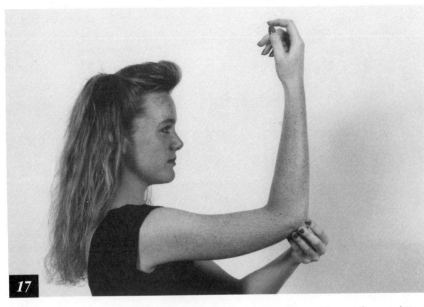

With the opposite hand, palm upward, support the opposite elbow with your fingers. (*Fig. 17*) Then gently but firmly flick the elbow (forearm) outward as you press the bones up into the joint. (*Fig. 18*)

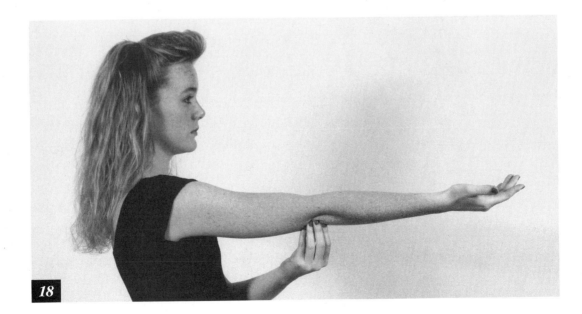

3 LATERAL ARM EXTENSION

This aligns the elbow joint laterally. Perform the lateral arm extension three times on each arm. Repeat the exercises on the opposite arm. This exercise can be done as often as needed to achieve desired results.

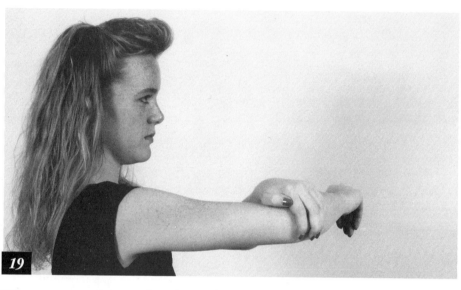

19

With your arm extended out in front of you, palm down, support the elbow joint. (*Fig. 19*) With opposite hand, bend the elbow, and flick the forearm outward as you firmly support the elbow joint. (*Fig. 20*)

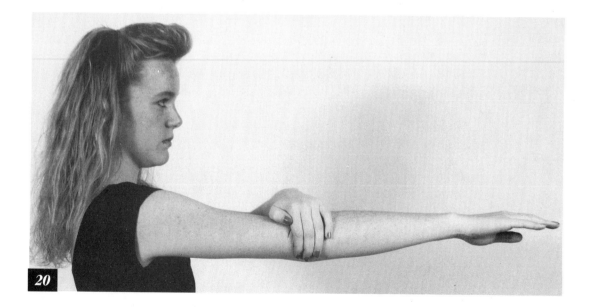

20

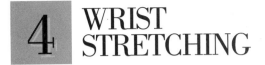

4 | WRIST STRETCHING

This stretches the muscles and tendons on the front of the hand at the wrist joint.

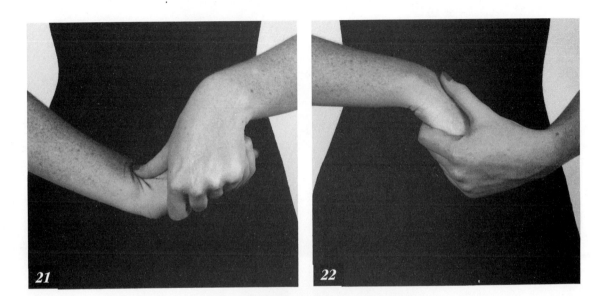

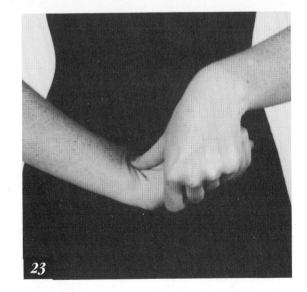

Place the thumb of the left hand on the top of the right wrist, thumb pointing toward the elbow and curl your fingers around the outer part of the right hand. (*Fig. 21*) This will support the right hand. Move the supported hand, flexing and extending it, (up and down) as you press the thumb into the wrist. (*Fig. 22*) Move the thumb slowly across the wrist, pressing into the tendons of the wrist, as you continue to flex and extend it. Perform this stretch three times. This can be repeated as often as needed.

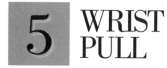

WRIST
PULL

This decreases the carpal tunnel and can give you relief from the pain. You may hear a popping sound of the bones shifting and realigning themselves. Not to worry, this is normal.

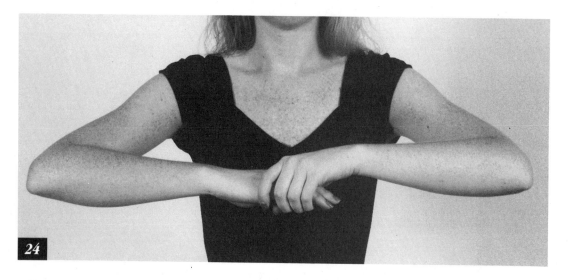

24

Shake the arm out and pull the hand away from the wrist. (*Fig. 24*).   Repeat on the opposite hand.

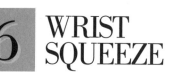

WRIST
SQUEEZE

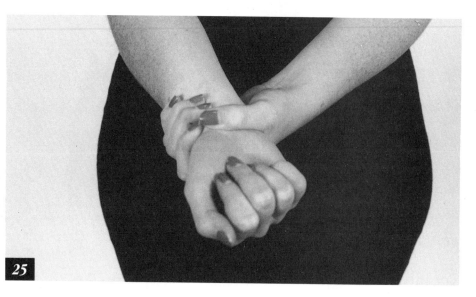

25

Then squeeze the wrist bones together gently but firmly. (*Fig. 25*).   This can be repeated as often as needed.
Repeat on the opposite hand.

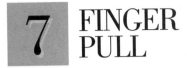

7 FINGER PULL

This will help to open up and restore the energy within the finger joints.

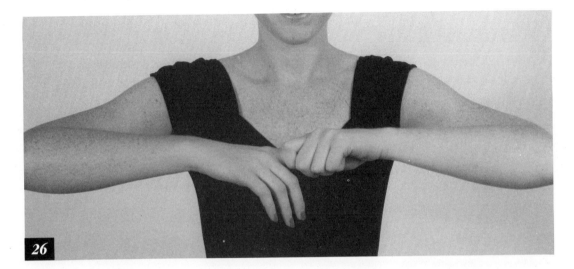

26

Gently grasp each finger at the base of the finger joint, closest to the hand (proximal end of the finger) and slowly pull. DO NOT JERK ON THE FINGERS. Once is enough. Repeat technique on the opposite hand. (*Fig. 26*).

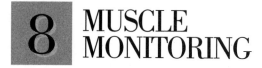

8 MUSCLE MONITORING

Repeat the muscle monitoring procedures Figs. 12, 13, 14. Check for increased strength of the thumb and little finger muscles and for grip strength, pg. 15. Repeat corrective techniques as many times as needed to get the desired results.

WORD OF CAUTION: Trauma to the hand and loss of its function is a serious matter. If after trying these simple techniques, no relief is evident, see a chiropractor specializing in applied kinesiology or a physician specializing in the hand for more indepth tests.

Corrective
Techniques

Prevention
Strength Exercises
& Stretches

IV.

All the exercises and stretches should be done slowly and with concentration. When strengthening the ligaments and tendons, light weights are recommended. NO MORE THAN 1-2 POUND WEIGHTS. The muscles will strengthen and tone also. The goal is to first strengthen the ligaments and tendons that hold the joints together. Do not overdo the exercises. The goal is to be able to do three sets of each exercise without pain or feeling sore. If after the second set of ten, your wrists are sore, stop. A slow building-up period of two-three months, using only light weights will strengthen the ligaments and tendons. Increase your weights accordingly. Stay consistent and the results will show. ▶

Doing these exercises daily, and correcting the joint alignment throughout the day as needed, will help you to maintain your wrist stability and avoid Carpal Tunnel Syndrome.

Exercises and stretches for the neck, shoulders, arms, wrists and hands are designed to help release tension, strengthen and tone the muscles, tendons and ligaments of these joints. ALL EXERCISES SHOULD BE DONE SLOWLY AND CONSISTENTLY TO ACHIEVE MAXIMUM RESULTS.

1 NECK EXERCISES
Checking Range of Motion

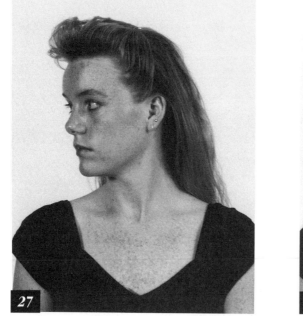

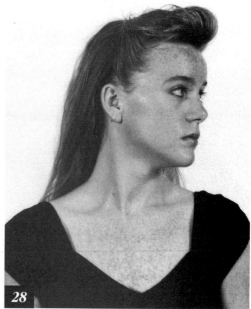

To check for range of motion of the neck, first turn the head to the right, then turn to the left. Feel the difference in muscle tightness between the two sides. Begin the exercises for both the shoulder and the neck. At the completion of the exercises, check to see if the range of motion has improved and the tightness in the neck and shoulders has decreased. (*Fig. 27 & 28*).

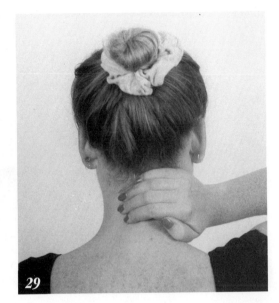

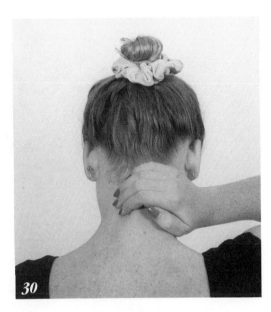

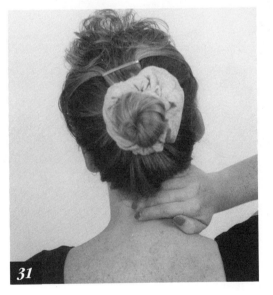

Place the hand, palm down, over the back of the neck. Firmly press your fingertips along the edge of the neck vertebrae and squeeze the neck muscles. Maintain firm pressure as you move the head forwards and backwards. Perform this exercise slowly, ten times. Relax and breathe slowly and deeply. Repeat exercise on opposite side of the neck. (*Fig. 29, 30 & 31*).

3 | NECK EXERCISES
Isometric Stretch

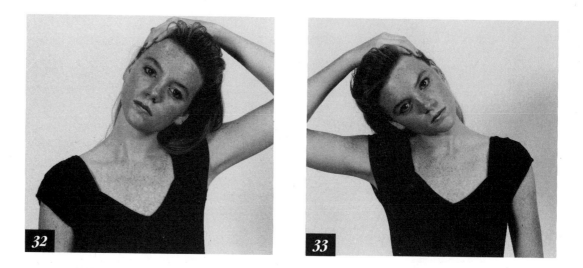

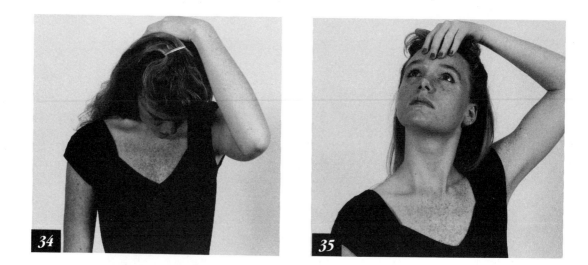

Isometric exercises performed in range of motion (head moves forward, backward, and to each side) help to strengthen and stretch the muscles, tendons and ligaments of the neck. (*Fig. 32, 33 & 34*).

As in *Fig. 32, 33, 34 & 35* place the hand on the side of the head. Inhale. On the Exhale, gently push into your hand ten percent of your strength for a five second count. Release. Slowly stretch the neck a little farther in the direction of range of motion of the neck. Repeat the stretch three times in each direction. DO NOT PULL ON THE NECK. ONLY GO AS FAR AS IT IS COMFORTABLE.

4 SHOULDER EXERCISES
Shoulder Half-Circles

This will help to release tension in the shoulder muscles and increase range of motion.

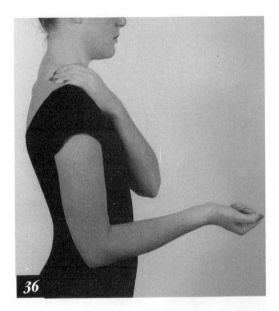

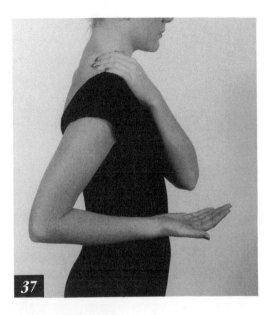

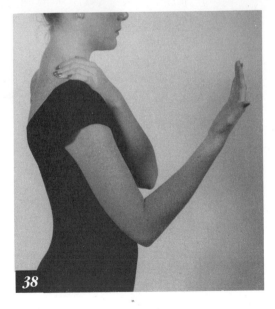

Standing or sitting, bend the elbow to 90 degrees and hold it close to the body. With the opposite hand, firmly press your fingertips into the shoulder muscle as you move your arm forward and backward. Maintain pressure at all times throughout the movement. Perform this slowly, ten times.

Perform the exercise on the opposite shoulder. Relax and breathe slowly and deeply. Repeat this exercise as often as needed. (*Fig. 36, 37 & 38*).

SHOULDER EXERCISES
Shoulder Raises Full-Circles

This will help to release tension in the shoulder muscles and increase range of motion.

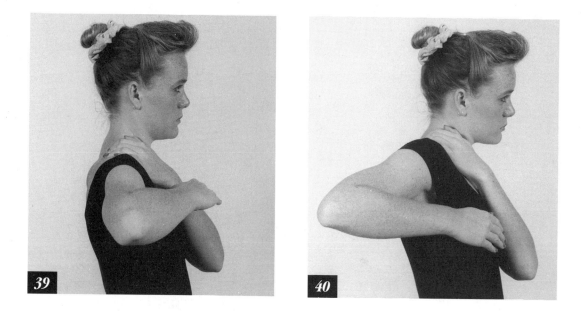

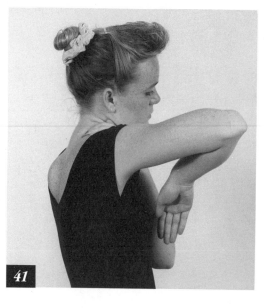

Standing or sitting, bend elbow and raise the arm to shoulder level. With the opposite hand, firmly press your fingertips into the shoulder muscle. Maintain a firm pressure as you move the arm in a clockwise direction. Continue to press into the shoulder muscle. Repeat in counter-clockwise direction. Perform this exercise ten times in each direction. Relax and breathe slowly and deeply. (*Fig. 39, 40 & 41*).

SHOULDER EXERCISES
Shoulder Shakes

This will help to relax the shoulder muscles.

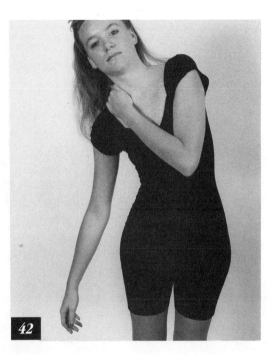

42

Take the opposite hand to the opposite shoulder-grab hold of the shoulder muscle (Trapezius m.), lean over to the side and shake the arm hanging down. Hold pressure on the shoulder muscle for a 10 second count. Relax and breathe slowly and deeply. Repeat on the opposite shoulder. Repeat as often as needed. *(Fig. 42)*.

SHOULDER EXERCISES
Shoulder Shrugs

Inhale. Slowly raise the shoulders to the ears. Hold for a five second count. Exhale. Slowly lower the shoulders. Do this ten times. Breathe slowly and deeply. This will relax the shoulders and upper back.

SHOULDER EXERCISES
Shoulder Rolls

Slowly roll the shoulders forward. Reverse and roll the shoulders backward. Relax the facial muscles and breathe slowly and deeply. Perform this ten times in both directions. This will relax the shoulders and upper back.

9 SHOULDER STRETCHES
Shoulders, Chest and Elbow Stretch

*This stretch opens up the chest and shoulder area. *An added benefit is the extension of the elbow joint which helps in the realignment process.*

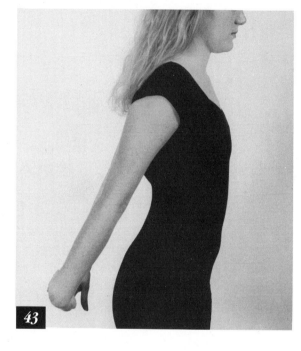

43

Standing, clasp, and interlace fingers together behind the back, palms toward back. Straighten the arms and elbows and stretch the arms up toward the sky and away from the back. Perform this slowly and hold the stretch for a ten second count. Relax and breathe slowly and deeply. Repeat this stretch as often as needed, especially if you find yourself slumping or rolling your shoulders forward. (*Fig. 43*).
*Only stretch as far as it is comfortable.

10 UPPER BACK STRETCH

Standing or seated. Clasp hands together. Extend arms out in front of you at chest level. Inhale. Exhale as you stretch forward, sinking the chest inward and rounding the shoulders forward (Imagine the chest caving in). Hold for five seconds. Breathe slowly and deeply. Inhale. Release the hands and draw the shoulders back and down. Repeat two-five times. This feels so good when the upper back is tired. *After performing this stretch, repeat #9.

11 | HAND EXERCISES
Ball Squeeze

This exercise will help to increase your grip strength.

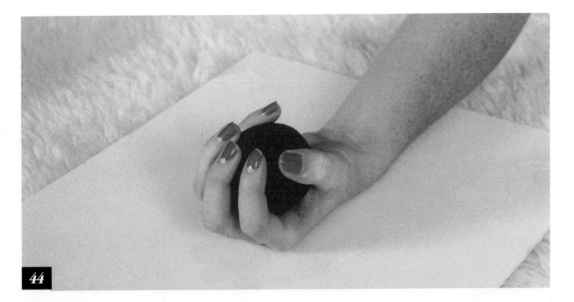

44

RUBBER BALL OR TENNIS BALL SQUEEZE - Start with one set of ten repetitions, two-three times a day. Squeeze slowly and firmly as long as there is no pain. Increase the number of sets of ten as you get stronger. (Fig. 44). Choose a soft, pliable rubber ball to start with. Move up to a tennis ball as you become stronger.

CHINESE EXERCISE BALLS - These two hollow chrome balls can be found in any natural health store. Rotate the balls in the palm of each hand to stimulate the energy in the fingers, acupuncture points and improve circulation of vital energy throughout the body. Rotate the balls ten times, two-three times a day. Increase the number of rotations as you become stronger. (Fig. 45).

32 ▶

Prevention

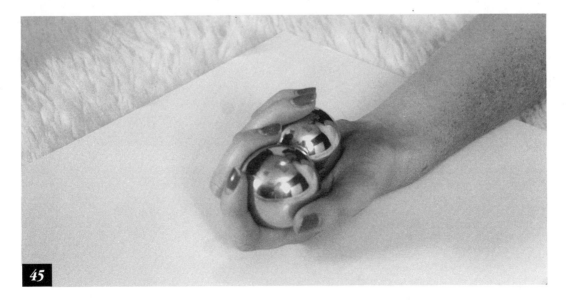

45

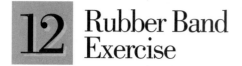 # Rubber Band Exercise

This exercise will help to increase the strength of the tendons and muscles in the hand and fingers.

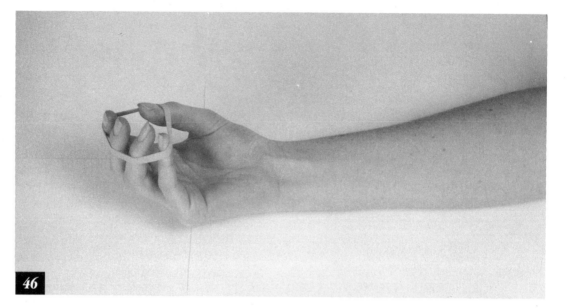

46

Place the rubber band around the fingers. Open and close the fingers. One set of ten repetitions, two-three times a day. Increase sets as your finger muscles become stronger. Increase the rubber tension of the band for increased resistance. (*Fig. 46 & 47*).

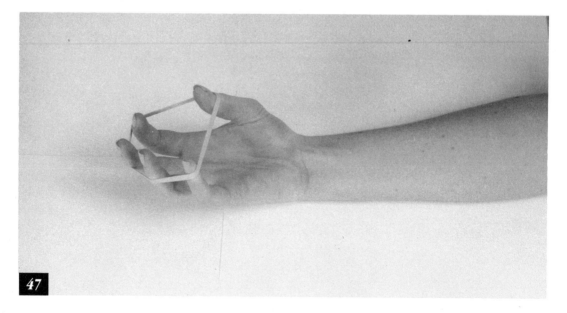

47

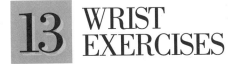

13 WRIST EXERCISES

All weight exercises should not be performed unless corrective techniques have been done first. Attempting to strengthen a misaligned joint with tight and sore muscles <u>will</u> <u>not</u> achieve the desired results*.

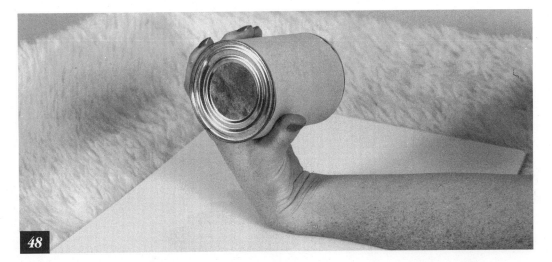

48

Using a one pound weight or 16 oz. can from the pantry:

I. FORWARD WRIST CURLS. Start with one set of ten repetitions, two-three times a day. Inhale. Exhale as you lift the weight. Lift and lower the weight slowly. Increase sets as you become stronger. Breathe slowly and deeply. (*Fig. 48*).

II. REVERSE WRIST CURLS. Start with one set of ten repetitions, two-three times a day. Inhale. Exhale as you lift the weight. Lift and lower the weight slowly. Increase sets as you become stronger. Breathe slowly and deeply. (*Fig. 49*).

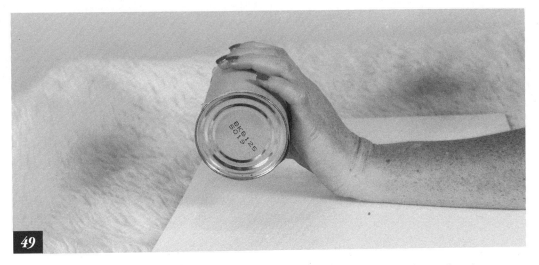

49

*Note: When strengthening tendons and ligaments you use light weights and increase the number of repetitions. Start slowly and be patient! Too much too soon, will deter your progress toward strong and stable joints.

14 ELBOW/UPPER ARM EXERCISES
Bicep Curls

These exercises are to help strengthen the upper arm muscles, biceps and triceps.

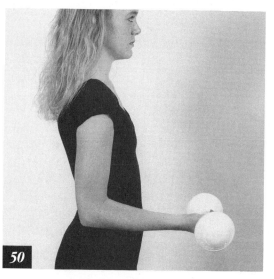

STARTING POSITION.

Using a two pound weight or one (32 oz.) can from the pantry:
Start with one set of ten repetitions, two-three times a day. Place the arm close to your side, elbow bent at a 90 degree angle. Inhale. Exhale as you slowly lift the weight. Inhale as you slowly lower the weight. Increase sets as you become stronger. Breathe slowly and deeply. . *(Fig. 50 & 51).*

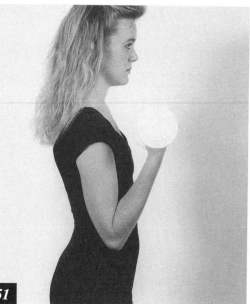

15 ELBOW/UPPER ARM EXERCISES
Tricep Curls.

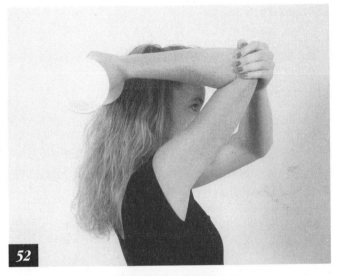

STARTING POSITION.

Raise the arm above the head, elbow bent with the forearm bent at a 90 degree angle to the shoulder (as pictured). The weight is resting in the hand. Opposite hand supports the elbow. Inhale. Exhale as you slowly lift the weight toward the sky. Inhale as you slowly lower the weight. Breathe slowly and deeply. ALWAYS SUPPORT THE ELBOW JOINT. Start with one set of ten repetitions, two-three times a day. Increase sets as you become stronger. *This recommendation is for the person who has never done any weight training before. If you go too fast in your training, tendinitis can develop. (*Fig. 52 & 53*).

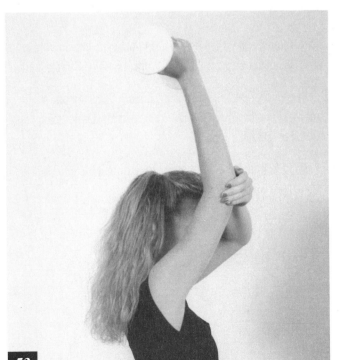

16 RANGE OF MOTION (ROM) EXERCISES AND STRETCHES FOR THE HANDS.

Begin the day with these warm up exercises. They are designed to increase range of motion, glide of the tendons, and stretch the muscles of the hands and fingers. They can be performed anytime and anywhere.

1. Hand Circles: Clockwise and counterclockwise circles. Five times each direction.

2. Fist Clinches: Open and close your fists rapidly five times.

3. Wrist Bends: Stretch the wrists forward and backward. Hold for a four second count in each direction. Use the opposite hand to help perform the exercise.

4. Finger Bends: Stretch fingers forward and backward, one at a time. Hold for a one-two second count. Use the opposite hand to help perform the exercise.

5. Finger Rotations: Rotate the fingers clockwise and counterclockwise. Use the opposite hand to help perform the exercise.

6. Finger Pulls: Pull gently on the fingers, grasping the finger joint closest to the hand.

7. Hand Shakes: Shake hands gently.

8. Finger Spread: Spread your fingers wide apart and stretch fingers outward.

9. Finger/Thumb Touch to the Palm: Individually, touch the pads of the fingers and thumb to the palm of the hand. You should be able to touch the pads to the palm of your hand easily.

10. Finger Touch to the Thumb: Individually, touch the pads of the fingers to the thumb. You should be able to touch the pads of the fingers to the thumb easily.

11. Finger-Joint Bends: Holding the tip of the finger, individually bend each joint of the finger. Repeat with each finger. Do not force a joint to bend. Work gradually with the joint to increase flexibility.

12. Finger Pinch: Pinch the ends of the fingers, firmly for one second count. Stimulates the energy in six meridians in the Chinese Acupuncture system. (Lung, Heart, Large Intestine, Small Intestine, Triple Heater and Pericardium.)

13. Palm Rub: Rub the palms together rapidly for a friction rub. Then massage the hands and fingers. A good way to increase circulation. This feels great!

Massage Therapy For The Arms And Hands

V.

Massage Therapy is a KEY COMPONENT in the prevention of Carpal Tunnel Syndrome!

To date, there are thousands of people who have had carpal tunnel surgery and many who have had multiple surgeries to try and correct this condition. The statistics for worker's compensation claims are mounting annually. There are two things all Carpal Tunnel patients have in common: 1. Extremely sore muscles, and 2. Scar tissue in the postsurgical area. Prior to surgery, the muscles of the arms and hands are tight, sore and have many trigger points. With each surgery, this is compounded. Muscle spasms and scar tissue can reduce the movement, flexibility, and grip strength in the arms and hands, and create tremendous pain. ▶

38 ▶
Massage
Therapy
For The
Arms And
Hands

To release the muscle spasms, dissolve and smooth out the scar tissue, massage the muscles of the arms and hands. This will increase blood circulation that will provide nutrition to heal the tissues and restore nerve function. Massage the post-surgical site gently but firmly, gradually working deeper. If it is painful, massage a little lighter. Doing this several times a day speeds the healing process and recovery time. Even if it has been many years since surgery, this therapy still works.

I also suggest massaging with my Herbal Healing Balm. The herbs used in the balm are specific for healing injured tissues. (Refer to the back of the book for information on the Herbal Healing Balm.)

Massage, in general, for the whole body will alleviate tightness and soreness in the muscles that support the skeletal structure. By releasing the tension in the muscles, you will feel calm, relaxed and less stressful. With proper massage, recovery time is shortened.

Self-Massage for the arms and hands will help relieve the tension and pain felt in the muscles due to repetitive movements. By pressing into the muscles you will locate the trigger points that cause pain in the muscles. Trigger point release and the three massage strokes described are easy to perform and can help relieve pain in the muscles of the arms and hands.

Massage
Therapy
For The
Arms And
Hands

TRIGGER POINT RELEASE AND MASSAGE STROKES FOR THE ARMS AND HANDS

1

Perform steps 1,2 3, and 4 in order to achieve the best results.

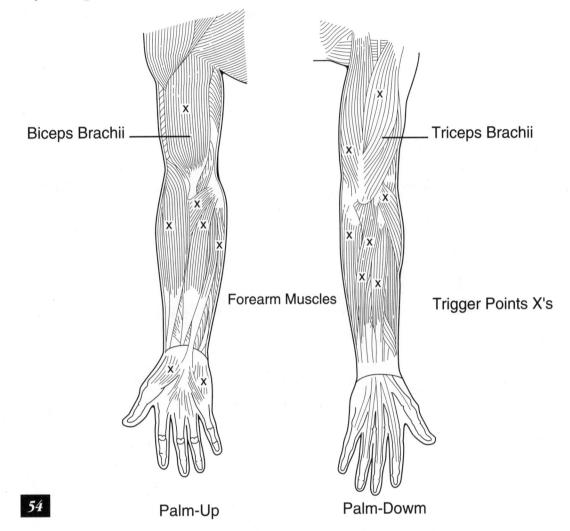

Biceps Brachii

Triceps Brachii

Forearm Muscles

Trigger Points X's

Palm-Up

Palm-Dowm

54

40 ▶

Massage
Therapy
For The
Arms And
Hands

#1. TRIGGER POINT RELEASE- A trigger point is a hypersensitive area in a muscle that is tender to the touch. They are found throughout the body's musculature. A trigger point may become more active when physical or emotional stress or trauma is inflicted upon the body. When it "fires" it sets off a continuous cycle of spasm and pain. The muscles become tighter and contract when overworked and overstrained, such as in repetitive hand movements. The forearm and hand muscles begin to fatigue and the "muscle energy" in the muscle decreases. (Example: Unplugging the electrical cord from the wall current). As the muscles become tighter, more and more trigger points are activated, the spasm/pain cycle intensifies and the muscles loose mobility and refuse to work anymore.
A trigger point has a referral area of pain. The pain from a trigger point may radiate to another area of the arm. To locate a trigger point, press into the muscle. If there is pain, you have located a trigger point. The muscles will feel tight, ropy and elicit pain at the touch of your fingertips. Hold firm pressure in that area, up to 90 seconds or longer, relax and breathe slowly and deeply, until you feel the pain begin to dissipate. Then lightly massage it and move on to another area in the muscle. The release of the trigger points along with massage therapy will allow the muscle fibers to lengthen and relax, lessening the tension and stress on the joints of the arm. (*Fig. 54*).

*For more information on trigger points refer to Pain Erasure, *The Bonnie Prudden Way*, by Bonnie Prudden.

MASSAGE STROKES
Cross Fiber Stroke

This stroke is a more specific stroke for a smaller area of the muscle. It is designed to breakdown and smooth out scar tissue, while increasing blood circulation and nutrition to the muscle.

41 ▶

Massage
Therapy
For The
Arms And
Hands

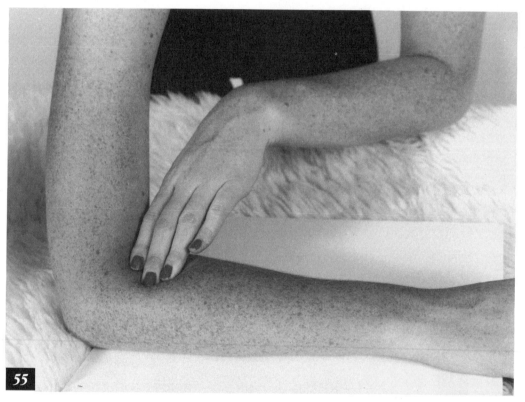

55

Place the fingertips on the arm muscle closest to the joint of the elbow. Gently but firmly press down into the muscle. Move the fingertips back and forth in a "sawing" motion. Repeat this movement in small areas of the muscle as you move up and down the length of the arm muscle. (*Fig. 55*).

3 MASSAGE STROKES
Broad Cross Fiber Stroke

This stroke is designed to cover a broader area of the muscle at one time. Its purpose is to unweave and smooth out a ropy muscle*, increase circulation and nutrition, flexibility and suppleness.

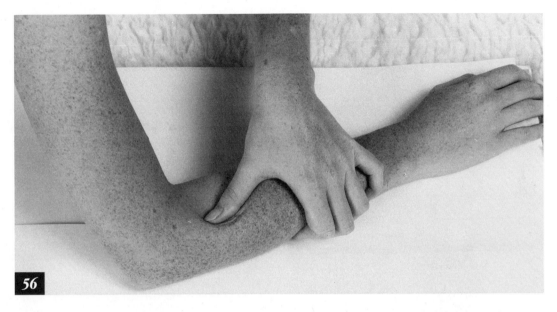

56

With the thumb pointing toward the elbow, gently but firmly press into the muscle as you massage across the muscle. Repeat this motion up and down the length of the arm. (*Fig. 56*).

*A ropy muscle feels like a tight guitar string when you massage against the fibers of the muscle.

42 ▶

Massage
Therapy
For The
Arms And
Hands

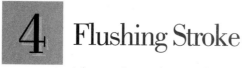

4 Flushing Stroke

This stroke is designed to push the blood and lymph toward the heart.

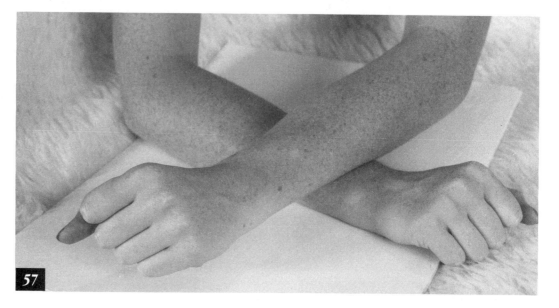

57

43 ▶

**Massage
Therapy
For The
Arms And
Hands**

With the forearm, gently but firmly press into the muscle and massage toward the heart. (*Fig. 57 & 58*). Note: ALWAYS STROKE TOWARD THE HEART TO EMPTY THE METABOLIC WASTE PRODUCTS INTO THE MAIN LYMPHATIC DUCTS FOR DRAINAGE.

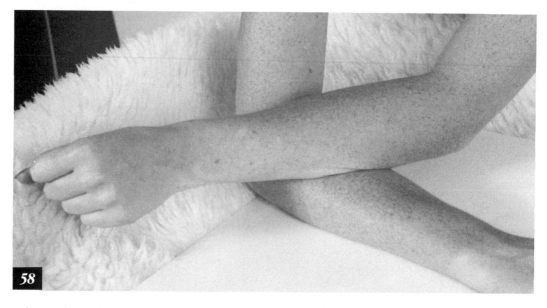

58

To locate a licensed massage therapist in your area, call the American Massage Therapy Association referral number for California, 1-800-696-2682, American Massage Therapy Association National number, 1-708-864-0123, and Associated Bodyworkers & Massage Professionals referral number 1-800-862-7724.

RECOMMENDED TREATMENT AND THERAPY

In most cases, Carpal Tunnel Syndrome or RSI is a structural and muscular disorder.

- *A person should seek consultation and assessment with a chiropractor specializing in applied kinesiology.*
- *With the exception of injury to the hand or arm, a physician specializing in the hand can rule out possibilities of a tumor, cyst, or nerve ganglion which can also cause pain and obstruction of the nerve pathway to the hand. Only in extreme cases where nerve dysfunction causes a loss of functional use of the arm and hand should surgery be considered.*
- *For the release of the muscles, a massage therapist can increase blood circulation, relax the muscles, release tension build-up, speed recovery time and relieve pain.*
- *For rehabilitation, a physical therapist can recommend exercises to strengthen the muscles of the neck, shoulders, arms and hands.*
- *Nutritional supplementation of Vitamin B6 is sometimes recommended for the relief of nerve, tendon and muscle inflammation in the elbow and wrist. Check with your doctor or chiropractor about this vitamin therapy.*

Past and present car accidents and traumas to the body, can all impede the neural transmission that give you the muscular strength needed to perform your daily activities.

The stability of the skeletal structure and the release of muscular tension and spasms is a must if Carpal Tunnel Syndrome or RSI injuries are to be corrected and prevented.

> WORD OF CAUTION: Trauma to the hand and loss of its function is a serious matter. If after trying these simple techniques, no relief is evident, see a chiropractor specializing in applied kinesiology or a physician specializing in the hand for more indepth tests.

44 ▶

Massage
Therapy
For The
Arms And
Hands

HERBAL HEALING BALM

The herbs in the Healing Balm have been extracted from ten herbs. In addition, it includes nine other ingredients that aid in the healing process of injured tissue. Use only a small amount of the balm. It goes a long way.

HERBS AND WHAT THEY DO

BLACK WALNUT LEAVES: Astringent

CHAPARRAL: Antiseptic

COMFREY LEAF AND ROOT: Demulcent, Vulnerary, Astringent

LOBELIA: Antispasmodic

MARSHMALLOW: Demulcent, Emollient, Vulnerary

MULLEIN LEAF: Astringent, Vulnerary, Demulcent

SKULLCAP: Antispasmodic

WHITE OAK BARK : Astringent

WORMWOOD: Antiseptic

GRAVEL ROOT: Astringent, Antiseptic, Demulcent

ADDED INGREDIENTS:

ST. JOHNS WART OIL: Stimulates circulation and restores local neural transmission.

ARNICA OIL: Curative, promotes cell growth and wound healing.

WINTERGREEN OIL: Pain relief; warms and relaxes the muscles.

CEDAR LEAF OIL: Stimulates circulation, warms and relaxes the muscles, pain relief, local disinfectant, and anti-inflammatory.

CASTOR OIL: Stimulates the local lymphatic circulation and draws out toxins from the tissues.

CITRICIDAL: (Grapefruit seed extract) - bacterialcidal and a local disinfectant.

BEESWAX: Softens the tissues.

LANOLIN: Holds moisture in the tissues.

VEGETABLE GLYCERIN: Softens the tissues.

GLOSSARY OF PHARMACOLOGICAL TERMS

Antiseptic: Inhibits growth of micro-organisms.

Antispasmodic: Prevents or eases muscular spasms or convulsions.

Astringent: Causes contraction of tissues, checking the discharge of fluid and mucus. Generally antiseptic.

Demulcent: Soothes inflamed mucus surfaces and protects them from irritation. Cools, coats and lubricates.

Emollient: Softens the tissues.

Vulnerary: Curative, promotes cell growth and wound healing.

Massage Therapy For The Arms And Hands

In my practice, I massage the Herbal Healing Balm into sore and tight muscles to help with the pain and muscular spasms created by repetitive movements. By working the balm into the muscle tissue, adhesions smooth out, the muscles relax and the pain slowly subsides. It can also be used to heal open cuts and scrapes. It is a great addition to any first aid kit!

To Order the Herbal Healing Balm:
Write Sports Touch®
P.O. Box 221074
San Diego, CA 92192-1074
Tel.: (619) 455-5283
Fax: (619) 455-5039

Acupressure Points For The Hand

VI.

Acupressure, a non-invasive form of Acupuncture, is practiced by applying pressure at points along the fourteen meridian channels or energy pathways. By pressing on these points, it is possible to release "Blocked Energy," which can then flow fluidly throughout the body to relieve pain and muscle soreness. By using these specific points for the hand, you can restore vital energy, strength and circulation. ▶

1 LARGE INTESTINE 4

For the relief of contracture and pain in the arms, hands and fingers. Relief of pain involving strains and sprains. Moves blood and energy.

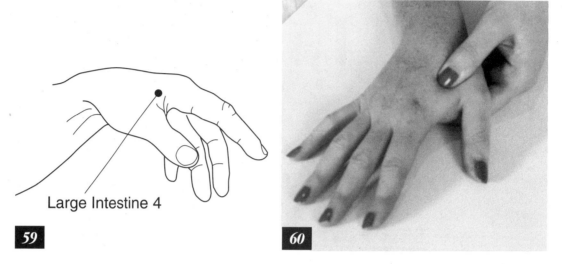

Large Intestine 4

59

60

Locate point in the middle of the web between the thumb and second finger. Press and rub firmly for 10-30 seconds or as long as needed to achieve desired results. Relax and breathe slowly and deeply. (*Fig. 59 & 60*)

2 BAXIE POINTS

For the relief of spasms and contracture in the muscles of the hand. Increases circulation, decreases swelling.

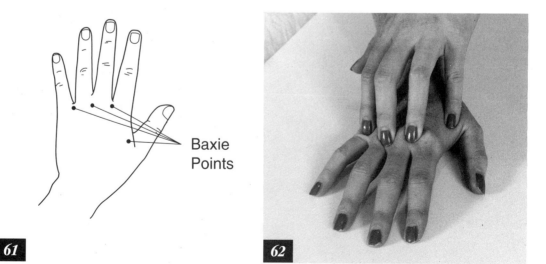

Baxie
Points

61

62

Locate points on the top of the hand, between the knuckles on the hand, at the beginning of the fingers. Press and rub firmly for 10-30 seconds or as long as needed to achieve desired results. Relax and breathe slowly and deeply. (*Fig.61 & 62*)

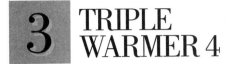

3 TRIPLE WARMER 4

Increases energy. Relieves pain in the shoulder, arm, wrist and hand.

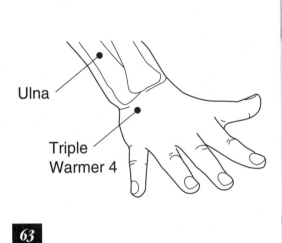

Ulna

Triple
Warmer 4

63

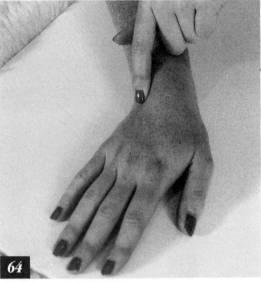

64

Locate point on the top of the hand, little finger side, in the crease of the wrist in front of the ulna bone. (This bone protrudes up). Press and rub firmly for 10-30 seconds or as long as needed to achieve desired results. Relax and breathe slowly and deeply. (*Fig. 63 & 64*)

PERICARDIUM 6

For the relief of pain and contracture in the elbow and the arm.

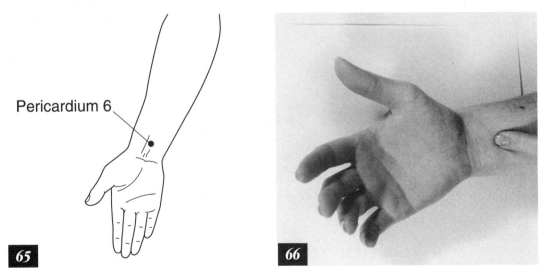

Pericardium 6

65

66

Locate point on the inside of the forearm, two fingers from the crease of the wrist, in the center of the forearm, between the tendons. Press and rub firmly for 10-30 seconds or as long as needed to achieve desired results. Relax and breathe slowly and deeply. (*Fig. 65 & 66*)

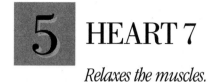

5 HEART 7

Relaxes the muscles.

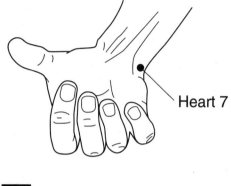

Heart 7

67

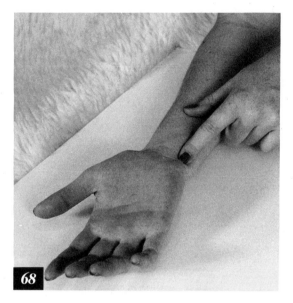

68

Locate point on the inside of the forearm, little finger side, in the crease of the wrist, at the junction of the wrist and start of the hand. Hold lightly and gently massage. Breathe into this point slowly and deeply. Hold for as long as needed to achieve desired results. (*Fig. 67 & 68*)

The Lymphatic System

VII.

The lymphatic system is the cleansing system of the body. It plays a pivotal role in the body's defense mechanism against disease.

Frank Chapman, D.O., discovered the neurolymphatic reflex points in the 1930s. They are known as the "Chapman Reflexes." He correlated them with specific glands and organs. In the 1960s, George Goodheart, D.C., correlated the Chapman Reflexes with specific muscles. ▶

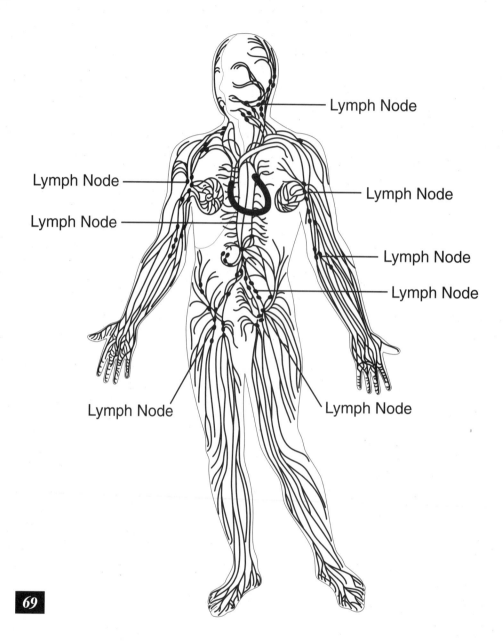

Lymph Node

Lymph Node

Lymph Node

Lymph Node

Lymph Node

Lymph Node

Lymph Node

Lymph Node

Lymph Node

69

The lymphatic system is known as the cleansing system of the body. It helps to filter out and dispose of metabolic waste products that accumulate in the body. The lymph system is continuously detoxifying the body and strengthening the immune system. It is composed of nodes that are made up of a network of vessels, capillaries and ducts. When we perform repetitive movements with our muscles, this is exercise. The arm and hand muscles are constantly moving and accumulating metabolic waste products which make our muscles feel sore, heavy and fatigued. Our lymph system is constantly flushing our muscles but sometimes it takes days before our muscles feel better. There is a solution to speed up this process. It is called Neurolymphatic Massage.

NEUROLYMPHATIC REFLEX POINTS FOR THE NECK, UPPER BACK, SHOULDERS, ARMS & HANDS

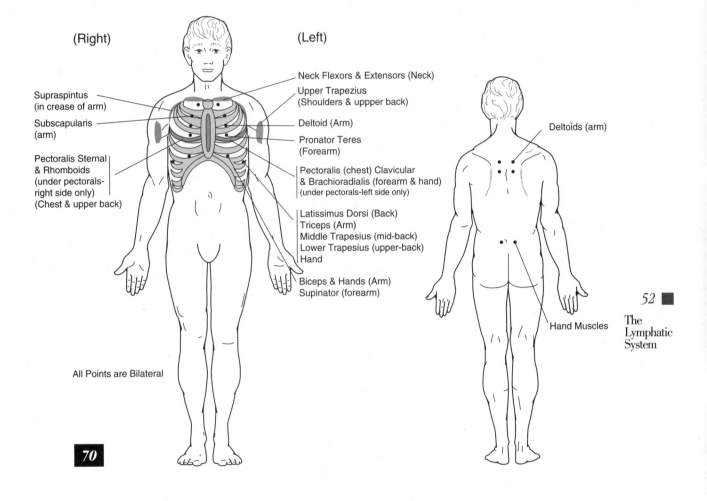

(Right)

Supraspintus
(in crease of arm)

Subscapularis
(arm)

Pectoralis Sternal
& Rhomboids
(under pectorals-
right side only)
(Chest & upper back)

All Points are Bilateral

70

(Left)

Neck Flexors & Extensors (Neck)

Upper Trapezius
(Shoulders & uppper back)

Deltoid (Arm)

Pronator Teres
(Forearm)

Pectoralis (chest) Clavicular
& Brachioradialis (forearm & hand)
(under pectorals-left side only)

Latissimus Dorsi (Back)
Triceps (Arm)
Middle Trapesius (mid-back)
Lower Trapesius (upper-back)
Hand

Biceps & Hands (Arm)
Supinator (forearm)

Deltoids (arm)

Hand Muscles

52
The
Lymphatic
System

Used within the system of Applied Kinesiology are neurolymphatic reflex points. They are called the "Chapman Reflexes." These are specific points and areas located on the front and back of the body that correlate muscles to the lymphatic system. Every muscle has an associated neurolymphatic reflex point. By rubbing these points firmly and deeply, one-five minutes, or as long as it is needed, you can alleviate the pain and soreness by decreasing the inflammation in the affected area. A healthy muscle will feel light, relaxed, flexible and supple. An overworked and overstrained muscle will feel heavy, sore, tight and painful to the touch.

Refer to the graphic for the location of the neurolymphatic reflex points for the neck, upper back, shoulders, arms and hands. (*Fig. 70*)

*Footnote: For more information on Neurolymphatic reflex points refer to Applied Kinesiology Synopsis by David S. Walther and Touch For Health by John Thie, D.C.

Ergonomics Of The Workplace

VIII.

Ergonomics is the science of how the body and the workstation equipment (chair, desk height, etc.) is adjusted to fit the body. ▶

53 ▶
Ergonomics
Of The
Workplace

In today's workplace, correct postural alignment of the body is necessary to avoid the physical aches and pains that come from using improper equipment to support the physical structure. Businesses spend thousands of dollars a year on ergonomically safe office equipment to insure the comfort of each employee. Even when the ergonomically sound equipment is in place, the employee may have the same physical aches and pains. Ergonomics is a necessary part of a good workstation, but it is only part of the solution to solve the cause of the problem.

You can spend thousands of dollars on the best bicycle, but it won't help you get up the hill any faster if you don't invest in the maintenance of the Body. There is no protocol for the human body in the standards set for ergonomics.

Everyday people work at jobs that require them to sit for long hours, push file drawers, bend, lift, and stoop. After a number of years, these positions and movements begin to take there toll on the body. Low back and neck pain, hip and leg pain, hand and wrist pain, shoulder and elbow pain, and foot pain become the complaints most often heard by employers. The employee is using his/her muscles just like an athlete but in very specific movements as it relates to the job. The stress on the body's muscles can cause tightness and soreness, create trigger points (see glossary) and eventually become very painful. Loss of function and decreased mobility are the result.

The feeling of "old age" does not have to become a reality if you incorporate preventive therapies into your daily life. My recipe for preventing old age is as follows: 1. Regular chiropractic, once or twice a month, insures the stability of the skeletal structure. 2. Massage therapy, in my opinion, is the key component to keeping the body free of stress and pain. Massage therapy is not a luxury, it is a necessity! Once a week or twice a month is suggested to help maintain flexibility and mobility and restore and maintain normal muscular functions. 3. Acupuncture, once or twice a month, helps maintain the balance of vital energy and harmony throughout the body. 4. A balanced nutritional program. 5. Exercise. 6. Plenty of rest, relaxation, and laughter!

The body is a magnificent machine given to us through the grace of God. If you take care of it and don't wait until it is in pain and becomes sick, it will last a long time.

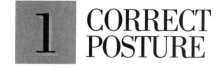

1 CORRECT POSTURE

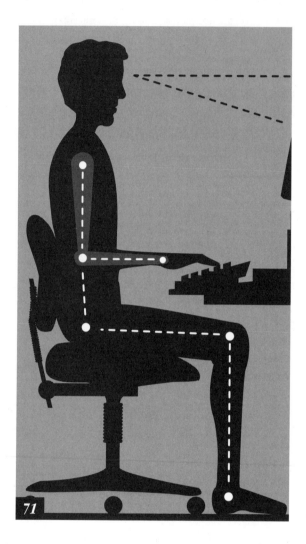

Correct Posture at a workstation starts with sitting up straight with proper support along the spinal curve. 1. BACK tilts slightly backward to increase the space between the torso and the thighs; thighs are at right angles to the torso. 2. SHOULDERS are down and slightly backward, stress free. 3. ARMS are relaxed. 4. FOREARMS are at right angles to the floor. 5. WRISTS and HANDS are in a neutral position, supported and slightly elevated. 6. FEET should be flat on the floor or on a footrest. 7. HEAD should be erect with the eyes directed slightly down (approximately 15° below the horizon) to view the computer screen.

Correct posture allows for increased blood flow throughout the body and reduces spinal compression.

2 CORRECT AND INCORRECT POSTURE
Aggravating Your Wrist

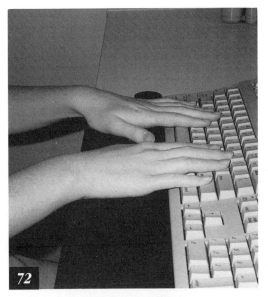

NEUTRAL POSITION
The wrist joints are parallel to the ground.

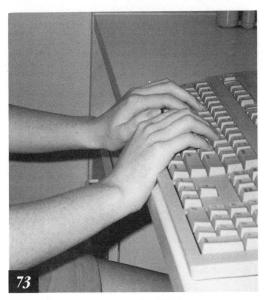

HYPEREXTENSION

At work, try to avoid putting your hands in compromising positions that can aggravate your arm and wrist joints. For example, a computer operator who sits and types all day and does not properly support the wrist joints may experience numbness and tingling due to hyperextension of the wrist joint. Placing a three-quarter inch foam pad in front of the keyboard will reduce this problem. *(Fig. 72 & 73).*

3 INCORRECT POSTURE
Habitual Backward Bending

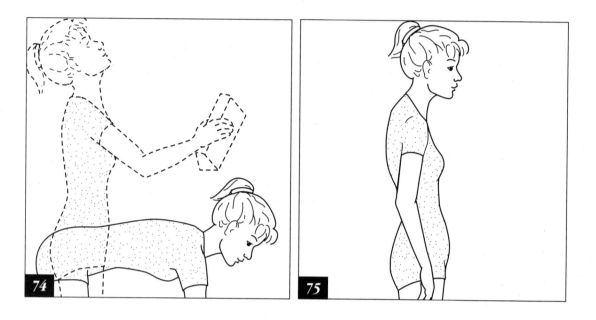

Ergonomics
Of The
Workplace

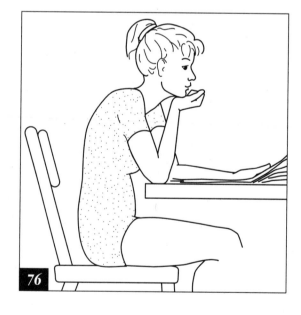

Demonstrates habitual backward bending of the neck and how postural habits acquired at home or at work can cause recurrent minor injury to the joints of the neck. Continual irritation can inflame the nerve root, causing pain in the neck, shoulders, arms and hands. *(Fig. 74, 75 & 76)*

INCORRECT POSTURE
Habitual Forward Neck Bending

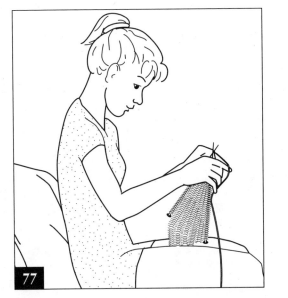

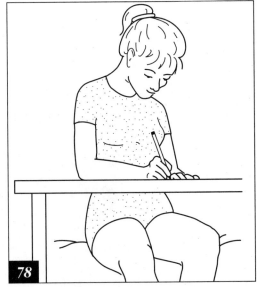

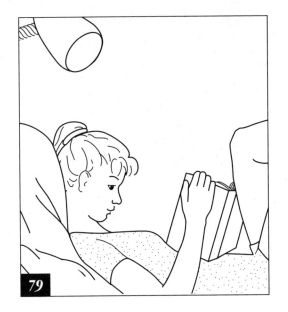

Demonstrates the constant habit of forward neck bending. While this may seem harmless, continual irritation on the neck vertebrae can result in permanent damage to the nerves and spinal discs, contributing to headaches, numbness and tingling in the arms and hands, with possible shoulder weakness. (*Fig. 77, 78 & 79*).

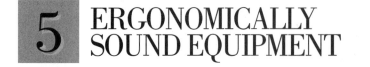

5 ERGONOMICALLY SOUND EQUIPMENT

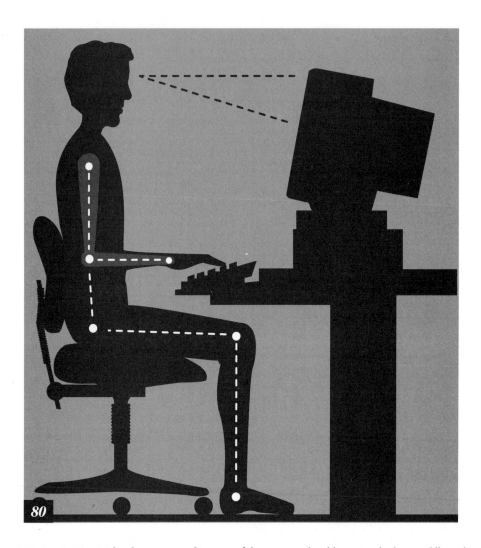

1. WELL-DESIGNED CHAIR. The chair protects the curve of the spine. It should support the low, middle and upper curve of the spine to prevent slouching. This reduces strain on the neck, shoulders, back, arms, hands, hips, legs and feet.

The chair should have an adjustable height and a tilt mechanism for the back and seat. A swivel option allows you to rotate your entire body, instead of twisting from the low back. Coasters on the legs of the chair allow you to move more easily, which decreases the stress on the legs and buttock muscles.

The use of arm rests create some debate. Some experts say they aggravate wrist problems and promote poor posture. Others find them a useful resting place to take the strain off the arms and hands.

2. STANDARD DESK HEIGHT. The desk should be at waist level, which can be determined by the height of the chair.

3. KEYBOARD ANGLE. The surface of the desk on which the keyboard rests should be arranged to maintain the wrist in a neutral position. In fig. 72, the wrist joints are flat and supported by a 3/4 inch pad that sits in front of the keyboard.

A study by the Labor Department reported turnover dropped to 5% a year from 35% a year after ergonomically designed workstations were installed. A NIOSH study showed a 24% increased in work performance at ergonomically designed workstations over traditional ones.

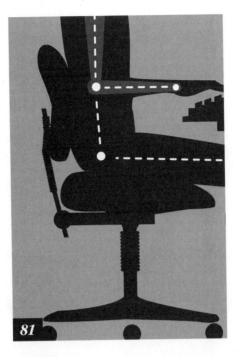

CHAIR-Back rest should fit the curve of the lower back. Seat inclines forward slightly to transfer pressure from the spine to the thighs and feet. Seat cushion bends downward at the front to relieve pressure on the thighs.

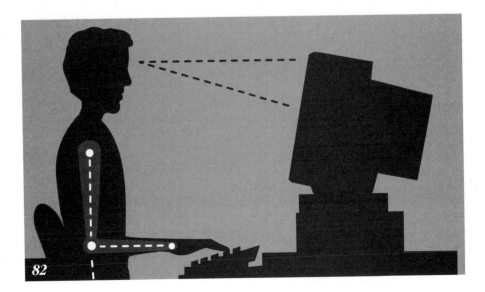

COMPUTER MONITOR-The top of the screen should be at eye level and the eyes cast down slightly to see the center of the screen.

Carpal Tunnel Ritual Index

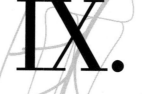

IX.

This is a brief overview of the book. Tips for the computer programmer, musician, weightlifter, golfer and for the tennis enthusiast. ▶

1. Correct posture. Sit up straight and tall. Chapter VIII. Pgs. 53-60, fig. 71.

2. Neck Massage - Pg. 17, figs. 15-16.

3. Neck Exercises and Stretches - Pgs. 25-27, figs. 27-35.

4. Shoulder Exercises and Stretches - Pgs. 28-31, figs. 36-43.

5. Elbow Joint - Self-correction..
   - Check grip strength, Pg. 15, fig. 14.
   - Forward alignment, Pg. 18, figs. 17-18.
   - Lateral alignment, Pg. 19, figs. 19-20.

6. Wrist Joint - Self-correction..
   - Wrist Stretch, Pg. 20, figs. 21-23.
   - Wrist Pull, Pg. 21, fig. 24.
   - Wrist Squeeze, Pg. 21, fig. 25.

7. Finger Pull. Gently but firmly pull the fingers to open up the finger joints. Pg. 22, fig. 26.

8. Acupressure Points. Press & Rub firmly. Chapter VI., Pgs. 46-49, figs. 59-68.

9. Neurolymphatic Reflex Points - Rub firmly the points for the neck, chest, back, arms and hands. Pg. 50, fig. 70.

10. Self-Massage the forearms and hands prior to work as a warm-up for the muscles. Receive a massage in the areas of the neck, chest, back, arms and hands. This will increase circulation, restore neural transmission and sensation and decrease the muscular tension throughout the upper body. A full body massage is recommended once a week or twice a month. To locate a licensed massage therapist, refer to Chapter V., Pgs. 38-43, figs. 54-58.

11. Perform a daily exercise program for the upper body and hands. Chapter IV., Pgs. 32-37, figs. 43-53.

12. Perform self-help exercises, 1-7 above throughout your daily routine. Steps 8, 9 & 10 can be done when needed. Refer to the Carpal Tunnel Syndrome/Prevention and Treatment for the procedures.

Tip: Computer Programmer - When you sit at a computer for extended hours, do 1-7 every two hours or as needed throughout your day.

Tip. Musician - perform warm-up exercises and self-massage the arms and hands prior to practice or performing. Perform the corrective exercises and stretches 1-10 before and after playing.

Warm-up Exercises:
   - Squeeze a rubber ball 10-20 times, both hands.
   - Rotate the Chinese Exercise Balls, 10 times in both hands.
   - Rubber Band exercise, 10-20 times, both hands.

Tip: Weightlifter - Perform steps 5-7 & 9 before and after a lift that involves any hyperflexion on the wrists. (i.e. flat bench press.)

Tip: Golfer - Perform steps 2-9 before you tee off. Steps 5-7 can be done throughout the game as needed. After the game, repeat steps 2-9.

Tip: Tennis - Perform steps 2-10 before the match. Steps 5-7 throughout the match as needed. Steps 5-7 & 9 after the match.

Every person, should receive a massage once a week to relieve stress, tension and pain, from the body; the athlete, for a more complete recovery from muscle soreness.

GLOSSARY

ABDUCTOR DIGITI MINIMI • Muscle on the little finger side, palm-side up. Abduction of little finger. Ulnar nerve innervation.

ABDUCTOR POLLICIS BREVIS • Muscle on thumb side, palm-side up. This muscle moves the thumb away from the palm. Median nerve innervation. Neurolymphatic reflex point under the left breast bone.

ADDUCTOR POLLICIS • Muscle on the thumb side, palm-side up. This muscle contributes to the power of grasp or holding on to objects. Ulnar nerve innervation. Neurolymphatic reflex point under the left breast bone.

APPLIED KINESIOLOGY • Study of movement of the muscles as applies to the evaluation of function.

ATROPHY • A wasting away due to nonuse. Example: a wasting away of the muscles (shrinking) and bone that surrounds a joint due to injury or disease.

BAXIE POINTS • Located on the hands, palm-side down between the webs of the five fingers. Relieves spasms and contracture of the muscles in the hands. Increases circulation and decreases swelling in the hands.

BICEPS BRACHII • Front arm muscle. Neurolymphatic reflex point is in the intercostal space between the 4th-5th ribs, three inches from the breastbone.

BLOCKED ENERGY • Energy not moving fluidly throughout the body. Example: Pain is blocked energy.

BRACHIORADIALIS • Forearm muscle. Flexes the elbow. Neurolymphatic reflex point is over the entire chest muscles.

DIABETES • A general term referring to disorders characterized by excessive urine excretion. A complication of diabetes is peripheral vascular disease.

DYNAMOMETER • An instrument that measures hand grip strength.

EXTENSION • The movement by which two ends of a jointed part are drawn away from each other. A straight line.

FLEXION • The movement of drawing two ends of a joint towards each other. The act of bending.

FLEXOR POLLICIS BREVIS • Muscle on the thumb, palm side-up. This muscle helps create flexion of the thumb. Median and ulnar nerve innervation. Neurolymphatic reflex point is under the left breast bone.

FLEXOR DIGITI MINIMI • Muscle on little finger, palm-side up. Flexion of little finger. Ulnar nerve innervation. Neurolymphatic reflex point is under the left breast bone.

HEART 7 • Located on the transverse crease of the wrist palm-side up, in the depression between the pisiform bone and the ulna bone, little finger side. For relaxation of all muscles.

HOOK OF HAMATE • Carpal or hand bone on the little finger side.

HYPEREXTENSION • Extreme bending backwards. Example: Bending wrist forward.

HYPERFLEXION • Extreme bending forwards. Example: Bending wrist backwards.

LARGE INTESTINE 4 • Located in the transverse crease, in the margin of the web between the thumb and index finger of the hand. Relieves contracture and pain in the fingers and the arms. Moves blood and energy.

LIGAMENT • A band of fibrous tissue that connects bones or cartilages, serving to support and strengthen the joints.

MEDIAN NERVE • Located down the midline of the forearm, palm-side up.

MERIDIAN CHANNEL • An energy pathway upon which the vital force of energy flows.

MISALIGNMENT • Not in a straight line. As referred to the bony structure of the body.

MYOPATHY • Any disease of the muscle.

NAVICULAR TUBEROSITY • A hand bone, thumb-side closest to the wrist.

NEURAL • Nerve.

NERVE GANGLION • A group of nerve cell bodies forming a knot like mass. A form of cystic tumor occurring on an aponeurosis or tendon, as in the wrist.

OPPONENS DIGITI MINIMI • Muscle on little finger side, palm-side up. Rotates the little finger to meet the thumb. Ulnar nerve innervation. Neurolymphatic reflex point is under the left breast bone.

OPPONENS DIGITI MINIMI • Muscle on little finger side, palm-side up. Rotates the little finger to meet the thumb. Ulnar nerve innervation. Neurolymphatic reflex point is under the left breast bone.

PERICARDIUM 6 • Located three fingers width from the crease of the wrist, between the tendon of muscles palmaris longus and muscle flexor carpi radialis. In the center of the arm, palm-side up. Relieves contracture and pain in the elbow and arm.

PHALENS TEST • A test to determine nerve entrapment. By bending the wrist in extreme backwards and forward movement.

PISIFORM BONE • A carpal or hand bone on the little finger side, closest to the wrist.

PRONATOR TERES • Wrist muscle. Innervated by the median nerve. Neurolymphatic reflex point is under left breast. Pronates the arm and flexes the elbow.

PRONATOR QUADRATUS • Wrist muscle. Innervated by the median nerve. Pronates the arm. Neurolymphatic reflex point is under the left breast.

PROXIMAL • Closer to any point of reference.

RADIUS BONE • A forearm bone located on the thumb side.

SUPINATOR • Arm muscle. Rotates the arm inward. Innervated by the radial nerve. Neurolymphatic reflex point is located underneath the left breast.

TENDINITIS • Inflamation of the tendon.

TINELS TEST • A test to determine nerve entrapment. By tapping the volar ligament over the median nerve to elicit a pain response.

TRICEPS BRACHII • Arm muscle. Extends the forearm. Innervated by the radial nerve. Neurolymphatic reflex point is located in the 7th intercostal space on the left, close to midline.

TRIGGER POINTS • A hypersensitive area in a muscle that is tender to the touch. Brought on by physical and emotional stress. When activated, a cycle of spasm and pain is set-up in the musculature.

TRIPLE WARMER 4 • Locate at the junction of the ulna and carpal bones in the depression lateral to the tendon of muscle extensor digitorum communis. Palm-side down, at the wrist junction, little finger side. For relief of pain in the wrist, arm and shoulder.

TRANSVERSE • Placed crosswise. At right angles. Example: Two bones at right angles to each other and a ligament stretched across them.

TUBERCLE OF TRAPEZIUM • A carpal or hand bone, thumb side in front of the NAVICULAR TUBEROSITY hand bone.

VITAL ENERGY • The motivating force that propels the body and provides the fuel for all the bodily functions.

VOLAR CARPAL LIGAMENT • A ligament that stretches across the transverse line of the wrist joint attaching to the carpal bones forming the carpal tunnel.

BIBLIOGRAPHY

Applied Kinesiology Synopsis, David S. Walther, Systems D.C, 1988.

Dorland's Illustrated Medical Dictionary, Twenty-five Edition, W.B. Saunders,1974.

Essentials of Chinese Acupuncture, First editions, Foreign Language Press, Bejing, China, 1980.

Illustrated Essentials of Musculoskeletal Anatomy, Kay W. Sieg and Sandra P. Adams, Megabooks, 1985.

Pain Erasure, The Bonnie Prudden Way, Bonnie Prudden, Ballantine Books, 1980.

Physical Examination of the Spine and Extremities, Stanley Hoppenfield, Appleton-Century Crofts, 1987.

Stevens, J. C., Sun, S., Beard, C. M., O'Fallon, W.M., Kurland, LT. Carpal Tunnel Syndrome in Rochester, Minnesota, 1961-1980. Neurology, 1988;38.

Sports Touch®/The Athletic Ritual, Kate Montgomery, Sports Touch®, 1990.

Touch For Health, John Thie, D.C., De Vorss and Company, Marina del Rey, California, 1979.

ADDITIONAL RESOURCES ON CARPAL TUNNEL SYNDROME

CARPAL TUNNEL SYNDROME & OVERVIEW. Crouch, Tammy

CARPAL TUNNEL SYNDROME. Pinsky, Mark A.

CARPAL TUNNEL SYNDROME, VOLUME XI, NEUROMUSCULAR CAUSES OF SPECIFIC PAIN PATTERNS. St. John, Paul

CTS, HOW TO RELIEVE AND PREVENT WRIST BURNOUT. Atencio, Rosemarie

NERVE COMPRESSION SYNDROMES, DIAGNOSIS AND TREATMENT. Szabo, Robert M. MD.

RELIEF FROM CARPAL TUNNEL SYNDROME. Tennenhaus, Norra

REPETITIVE STRAIN INJURY. Pascarelli, Emil

REPETITIVE STRAIN INJURY. Mill, Wendy

THE ULTIMATE HAND BOOK. Evans, Maja CMT, DH: Self-Care for Bodyworkers and Massage Therapists

FOR INFORMATION ON CARPAL TUNNEL SYNDROME ABSTRACTS FROM SCIENTIFIC RESEARCH FINDINGS:

Ragberg, M; Morgenstern, H; Kelsh M.
Impact of occupations and job tasks on the prevalence of carpal tunnel syndrome.
National Institute of Occupational Health, Division of Work and Environmental Physiology, Solina, Sweden
Scand J Work Environmental Health 1992, Dec. 18 (6):337-45
Unique Identifier: Medline 93134348

Moore, JS.
Carpal Tunnel Syndrome
Department of Preventive Medicine, Medical College of Wisconsin, Milwaukee, 53226.
Occup. Med., 1992, Oct.-Dec.; 7(4): 741-63
Unique Identifier: Medline 93031140

Weiss, AP; Akelman, E.
Carpal Tunnel Syndrome: a review
Department of Orthopedics, Brown University, Providence, RI.
RI Med. 1992, June; 75(6):303-6
Unique Identifier: Medline 9236487

Chiu KY; Ng WF; Wong WB; Choi CH; Chow SP.
Acute carpal tunnel syndrome caused by pseudogout.
Department of Orthopedic Surgery, University of Hong Kong, Queen Mary Hospital.
J Hand Surg. (Am) 1992 Mar; 17(2):299-302
Unique Identifier: Medline 92226436

Skandalakis, JE; Colborn, GL; Skandalakis, PN; McCollam SM; Skandalakis, LJ.
The Carpal Tunnel Syndrome: Part II.
Centers for Surgical Anatomy & Technique, Emory University, Atlanta, GA 30322.
Am Surg. 1992 Feb;58(2):77-81
Unique Identifier: Medline 92197911

Szabo, RM; Madison M.
Carpal Tunnel Syndrome
Department of Orthopedics, University of California, Davis, Sacramento.
Orthop Clin. North Am 1992 Jan;23(1):103-9
Unique Identifier: Medline 92107436

Mascola, JR; Rickman, LS.
Infectious causes of carpal tunnel syndrome: case report and review.
Infectious Diseases Division, National Naval Medical Center, Bethesda, Maryland.
Rev. Infect. Dis. 1991 Sept-Oct; 13(5):911-7.
Unique Identifier: Medline 92073810

Totten, PA; Hunter, JM.
Therapeutic techniques to enhance nerve gliding in thoracic outlet syndrome and carpal tunnel syndrome.
Hand Rehabilitation Center, Philadelphia, PA.
Hand Clin. 1991 Aug; 7(3):505-20.
Unique Identifier: Medline 92042332

Baker, EL; Ehrenberg, RL.
Preventing the work-related carpal tunnel syndrome: Physician reporting and diagnostic criteria.
National Institute for Occupational Safety and Health, Centers for Disease Control, Atlanta, GA 30333
Ann. Intern. Med. 1990 Mar. 1;112(5):317-9
Unique Identifier: Medline 90165116

Hunter, JM.
Recurrent carpal tunnel syndrome, epineural fibrous fixation, and traction neuropathy.
Jefferson Medical College, Thomas Jefferson University, Philadelphia, PA.
Hand Clin. 1991 Aug; 7(3):491-504
Unique Identifier: Medline 92042331

Kuschner, SH; Ebramzadeh, E; Johnson, D; Brien, WW; Sherman, R.
Tinel's sign and Phalen's test in carpal tunnel syndrome.
Department of Orthopedic Surgery, University of Southern California School of Medicine, Los Angeles, CA.
Orthopedics 1992 Nov:15(11):1297-302
Unique Identifier: Medline 93096704

SUPPORT GROUPS AND INFORMATION IN THE UNITED STATES

WE DO THE WORK
5867 Ocean View Drive
Oakland, CA 94618
(510) 547-8484
Provides a video tape on RSI about the problem as it exists in the workplace.

WORKSAFE TECHNOLOGIES INC.
15536 College Blvd.
Lenexa, KS 66219
W 913-492-8282, 913-492-2495 Fax
Denise Brown - President
Multi-discipline safety/injury prevention consulting firm for all companies who are experiencing work related injuries..

LABOR OCCUPATIONAL HEALTH PROGRAMS (LOHP)
Affiliated with University of California at Berkeley, School of Public Health
2525 Channing Way, 2nd Floor
Berkeley, CA 94720
510-642-5507
Resource library, interfaces with the unions, professionals, policy makers, employees, a
community service organization.
Robin Baker - Director

CARPAL TUNNEL SYNDROME/REPETITIVE STRAIN INJURY ASSOCIATION
A national and international non-profit association. Acts as a clearing house for information and support for
upper body extremity disorders. Perodic newsletter.
Stephanie Barnes - Director
P.O. Box 514
Santa Rosa, CA 95402
707-571-0397

COMPENSATION ALERT

A non-profit organization that educates, informs, and communicates with injured workers in all aspects.

Dorsey Hamilton - Director

Author of Basic Stuff, a primer on the California Workers Compensation system.

843 2nd Street

Santa Rosa, CA 95404

707-545-2266

JOB ACCOMMODATION NETWORK

Assists employers and employees in complying with the Americans with Disabilities Act.

West Virginia University

P.O. Box 6080

Morgantown, West Virginia, 26506-6080

1-800-526-7234

THE OFFICE TECHNOLOGY EDUCATION PROJECT

A Non-Profit Organization dedicated to the education and training of workers that suffer from arm/wrist and hand disorders in computer/office related work areas. Resource library/CTS support groups.

One Summer Street

Sommerville, MASS 02143

Erica Foldy - Executive director

617-776-2777

LABOR OCCUPATIONAL HEALTH PROGRAMS

Affiliated with University of California at Berkeley, School of Public Health. Resource library

Robing Baker - Director

2515 Channing Way, Second Floor

Berkeley, CA 94720

510-642-5507

SUPPORT GROUPS

SAN FRANCISCO BAY AREA SUPPORT
GROUPS NEWSLETTERS***

CTS/RSI Assoc. Newsletter Santa Rosa, CA.

Director: Stephanie Barnes.

707-571-0397

EAST BAY RSI SUPPORT GROUP.

3844 Ruby Street, Oakland, CA. 94609

Contact: Joan Lichterman

510-653-1802

SAN FRANCISCO RSI SUPPORT GROUP.
3101 California Street, #7
San Francisco, CA 94115
Contact: Judy Doane- H415-931-8780

SOUTH BAY RSI SUPPORT GROUP.
30 North Willard Ave. San Jose, CA 95126
Contact: Pat Rogge.
408-280-1134, Fax 408-294-2452

FREMONT RSI SUPPORT GROUP
42933 Hamilton Way
Fremont, CA 94538
Contact: Donna Chinn
W510-441-4289 (2-5)

FREMONT RSI SUPPORT GROUP
40554 Fremont Blvd.
Fremont, CA 94538
Contact: Leigh Strange
510-657-2201

FREMONT RSI SUPPORT GROUP
Hand Rehab. Associates
1999 Mowry Avenue, Ste. D-2
Fremont, CA 94538
Contact: Barbara Fong
W510-796-4263 (AM)

MARIN RSI SUPPORT GROUP
82 Rosewood Drive
Novato, CA 94947
Contact: Regina Schneider
415-898-5838H/415-989-8687W
Advice/Resources on Financial Assistance

MARIN RSI SUPPORT GROUP
582 Fernando Drive
Novato, CA 94945
Contact: Liza Smith
415-899-8040

SOUTH SAN FRANCISCO RSI SUPPORT GROUP
Caremark Peninsula Athletes Center
216 Mosswood Way
South San Francisco, CA 94080
Contact: Lynda Jensen
W415-589-0600

MORE TESTIMONIALS:

Two years ago my hands were numb about 50% of each day due to CARPAL TUNNEL SYN-DROME. Being a quilt maker and instructor, I knew I had to take measures to correct this. I was about to contact a surgeon when a friend suggested I call Kate Montgomery of San Diego, Calif. After talking to Kate, I ordered her book with much skepticism. After just one 10 minute session with her book I felt immediate relief. I continue to have relief when I work the simple hand exercises in her book. If I get careless and the symptoms return, I merely have to repeat the simple corrective techniques. I now tell every Quilter I come in contact with to get Kate's book before seeing a surgeon.

Lyn Mann

Quilt maker/Instructor

I am a career medical Transcriptionist who has seen many co-workers lose their ability to continue in their careers because of CTS and overuse syndrome.
The Forward Arm Extension (FAE) and the Lateral Arm Extensions (LAE), I couldn't help but notice, gave me immediate and really rather miraculous relief. Such simple movements. The miraculousness of the FAE and LAE sure give me confidence in the longer-term effects... Thanks again, Kate, for a great book.

Jane Daniel

Medical Transcriptionist

For six months I had been suffering with symptoms of carpal tunnel syndrome ... wore braces on both arms. This made my job extremely difficult and painful.
After a one hour session, I was amazed at the immediate relief I experienced. I walked around my house just touching everything ... the feeling had returned so quickly. When I returned to work the next day, it was as if nothing had ever been wrong with my hands. I was pain free!! Thanks Kate for giving me back my hands and arms and restoring my life to normal.

Julie-Rae Wilson

Data Processor

As a professional drummer, I became unable to play without wristbraces. Before meeting Kate Montgomery, I tried several different medical approaches. After just one visit to Kate, I was able to resume playing comfortably and my wrists were pain-free! As a professional drummer, my hands are my most valuable asset. Thanks to Kate Montgomery, I'll never suffer from wrist pain ever again!

Tyler Buckley
Professional Drummer

I have been a teacher of computer applications and a consultant for over ten years. During this time I have researched and taught my students ergonomics (proper posture, keyboard placement, etc.) strategies to prevent CTS. When I heard Kate speak and read her book, I saw a positive action that can be taken for both relief and prevention. So far, every person that I have shown Kate's seven step exercise to has experienced almost instant relief. I now teach the exercise and encourage my students to obtain Carpal Tunnel Syndrome/Prevention and Treatment for a permanent reference.

Howard Mayling
Computer Trainer

ACKNOWLEDGEMENTS

Thank you to my daughter Carissa for posing for the pictures. You have such patience! I love you.

To all my clients, Patti, Sheila, Cynthia, Jim, and many more, who have helped me to perfect my techniques for self-care, thank you.

Bill Lerner, D.C., for his contribution and knowledge on Carpal Tunnel Syndrome and his support.

Esther Platner, your support and friendship kept me going.

Rudy, thanks for a great remake!

Diane Gage for her editing and support.

Graham Smith for the use of your photography studio and patience.

John Finch, herbalist, for your wisdom and friendship.

Dr. Charles Lebo for his contribution on med-line research and Karen Perloth for her support.

A special thank you to Bo for her unwavering support and friendship and for sticking with me the last two years. Without you, this book would not be where it is today.

BIOGRAPHY

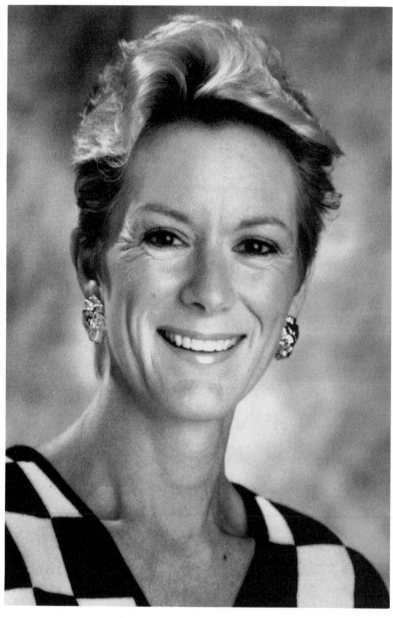

Kate Montgomery M.T., H.H.P., educator, healthcare consultant, certified Sports Massage Therapist, and Holistic Health Practitioner is versed in oriental medicine, sports massage and applied kinesiology. Over the last 21 years, Kate has taught her clients practical and functional techniques that improve and revitalize the body and mind. She is a frequent guests on numerous local, national and international radio and television programs.

KATE'S RECIPE FOR
A HEALTHY BODY!

1. Regular Chiropractic, insures a stable structure.

2. Massage Therapy, insures muscles free of stress, tension and pain.

3. Acupuncture, insures the balance of vital energy and harmony throughout the body.

4. A Balanced Nutritional Program, the right fuel strengthens the immune system.

5. A Daily Exercise and Stretching Program, to keep the body strong, flexible and mobile.

6. Meditation, to calm the mind and strengthen the spirit.

7. Plenty of Rest, Relaxation and Laughter!

With Love, Kate

PRICE LIST ORDER FORM

SPORTS TOUCH® INTERNATIONAL
Post Office Box 221074
San Diego, CA 92192-1074
Telephone (619) 455-5283
Facsimile (619) 455-5039

Prices Effective 5/1/94   Subject to change without notice

SOLD TO:

Name:_____

Address:_____

City:_____ State:_____ Zip:_____

Country:_____

Date Received:_____ Date Shipped:_____

Resale # If Applicable:_____

FORM OF PAYMENT:

Money Order   Check   Visa/MC/Amex

Visa/MC/Amex#:_____

Signature:_____

Telephone:_____

BOOKS

ITEMS	QUANTITY	COST/EACH	TOTAL
THE ATHLETIC RITUAL ISBN# 1-878069-00-4	_____ Book(s)	$24.95	$_____
A.R./W THERAPIST ADDENDUM *(For Massage Therapist and other Professionals)* ISBN# 1-878069-01-2	_____ Book(s)	$29.95	$_____
CARPAL TUNNEL SYNDROME ISBN# 1-878069-35-7	_____ Book(s)	$16.95	$_____

75 ■

Carpal
Tunnel
Ritual
Index

AUDIO/VIDEO

CARPAL TUNNEL SYNDROME - IF ONLY I KNEW... ISBN# 1-880688-03-4	_____ Audio(s)	$12.95	$_____
CARPAL TUNNEL SYNDROME - THE MONTGOMERY METHOD ISBN# 1-878069-05-5 (Due out in the Spring, '95)	_____ Video(s)	$29.95	$_____

HERBAL HEALING PRODUCTS

HERBAL HEALING COMPRESS	_____ Pack(s)	$10.00	$_____
HERBAL HEALING BALM (2oz.)	_____ Jar(s)	$16.00	$_____

PAYMENT

Please allow 2-4 weeks
For Delivery

Thank You, Kate

Total $_____
Discount %____ $_____
Subtotal $_____
(CA residents add sales tax) +Tax $_____
+Shipping & Handling $_____

TOTAL ORDER AMOUNT $_____

Please add $4.00 for the first order, $2.00 for additional item(s) for shipping and handling.